Dear

"You ... been my
one true friend -
rock - working
partner."

Journey
Into Health

Sheena Bull,
BSc. (Hons) Ag.

We have walked off miles
of stress and created love
for many years. Keep up
your fitness - forever
and have the life you deserve
I love you ♡ xoxo Sheena

◆ FriesenPress

Suite 300 - 990 Fort St
Victoria, BC, V8V 3K2
Canada

www.friesenpress.com

ISBN
978-1-4602-8950-1 (Hardcover)
978-1-4602-8951-8 (Paperback)
978-1-4602-8952-5 (eBook)

1. BIOGRAPHY & AUTOBIOGRAPHY, PERSONAL MEMOIRS

Distributed to the trade by The Ingram Book Company

Table of Contents

•

Introduction

My love affair with exercise began when I was fourteen and could not run a mile around the school track during a fitness test. I decided to start jogging regularly and by the end of a month of training, I took two and a half minutes off my time. That early success started my rewarding, exciting and sometimes tumultuous 35-year relationship with exercise.

My love affair with entrepreneurism began in my second year of university when I first perused the scholarship and bursary binder in the Dean's office, trying to find out which major would yield the greatest financial return. In the end, it turned out to be a minor in poultry science, which translated into almost ten thousand dollars of unclaimed scholarships and my name as a co-author of a paper published in the *American Poultry Science Journal*. My children were entertained for years with my poultry science stories. My clients would frequently comment on my university degree that I had framed and proudly displayed on a wall in my gym. "Bachelor of Science in Agriculture with a minor in Poultry Science?" they would ask with a certain hesitation. "It's completely compatible with being a personal trainer," I would reply with complete confidence. "Didn't you know that? Not to worry, you will understand after the first few workout sessions."

My two favorite activities were married together on Salt Spring Island fifteen years ago when I started a personal training studio in my home. It was a great way to run my own business while raising five active children. However, I felt that I was limiting myself by only working with clients one on one, and soon realized I was missing out on reaching a wider audience. Eventually, my desire to run a membership gym led me to sell my home and studio and embark on a complicated real estate journey with so much wheeling and dealing, that I began to feel like the female version of Donald Trump. Finally, in 2009, I was able to purchase a commercial building in Ganges on Salt Spring Island and start the membership gym I'd been hoping for. After months of careful planning and equipment selection, the doors were opened to the public to purchase monthly memberships. Alas – and in a rather spectacular anti-climax – no one came. Despite the fact that the only competitor on the island had equipment that had not been changed in over twenty years, no one made the switch to my clean, sleek, up-to-date gym. Those first few months were devastating, not to mention financially frightening.

Then I had a revelation. It was the kind of revelation you get when you remember where you put your car keys when you are certain you're going to miss the job interview. Or when you remember what your partner wanted for Christmas just before the shop sells out. Here on Salt Spring, there is a local joke that goes like this: "How many Salt Springers does it take to change a lightbulb?" Here's the answer: "Change!?!"

I realized that on our tiny island of ten thousand people who do not take easily to any kind of change, I was going to have to share with them the reasons *why* they should join this gym, instead of sharing *what* this gym is. That was the real beginning of my journey and where the real magic happened. Once we focused on the *why* instead of the *what*, the fitness studio went from zero members to 350 members and 70 personal training clients over the next three years. When the doors first opened, there was one personal trainer. Yes, it was yours truly. After two years, there was a team of four trainers.

The other gym in town proudly told everyone that their membership had not changed with the opening of a new club on the island, which means that 350 new customers had stepped forward to join my gym. With the increase in membership, what I came to realize is that the process of joining a gym is unique to each individual. It also became apparent to me how important it was that more people within a community join a gym and use the facility regularly as it promotes fitness and a greater sense of general wellbeing.

The Seven Reasons People Join a Gym

People join a gym for various reasons, but some of the more common reasons are below.

Inspiration—For many people, beginning to exercise is not fun or exciting. They may have motivations for going to the gym, such as wanting to look good for their tenth high school reunion or getting fit in order to get off certain medications, but they need inspiration to deeply stir something within them to be inspired to go to the gym. When they visit the website for a gym, they want to be inspired to take the action of joining a gym. It's human nature to need something that *comes from within* that causes people to rise up and do something.

It's hard to be inspired to run on a treadmill that is tucked into the corner of the laundry room. It's equally hard to be inspired to lift weights at home with the phone ringing and children using your equipment to build a fort. It's inspiration that gets you back to the gym for a spin class at seven o'clock in the morning or for that leg work out that you know you'll feel the next day.

Equipment—Another reason people join a gym is because of the equipment. It really is almost impossible to duplicate a gym in your home. Cleaning and maintenance are one less thing you have to think about when you hit your club for a workout. There are a wide variety of exercises available with the selection of equipment found at fitness facilities. The more diverse the exercise equipment, the less likely you are to become bored, lose motivation, or suffer overuse injuries from the excessive repetition of the same movements.

Community—Don't overlook the sense of community a gym provides. Once someone starts going to a gym, they quickly develop relationships with the staff and other members. This type of connection is healthy on many levels. Humans are social beings and need face to face connections. With advances in technology, it has become easier to hibernate and lose that connection that is essential for health and vitality. Gyms, by their very nature, serve to connect. They are all-inclusive clubs that span generations and bring diverse groups of people together around the common goal of health and fitness.

Expert Advice—When people join a gym they are looking for expert advice. They want assistance in developing an exercise program that suits their needs. When they have questions or concerns regarding exercise, most gym members rely on the expertise of the staff. My experience has taught me the absolute importance of consultation and guidance for gym members, particularly those individuals new to exercise. Having the expertise to rely on is often the difference between success and failure for many members.

Motivation—Most people need to be motivated to keep going to the gym. Inspiration is needed to find your way to the gym, but motivation is what keeps you coming back, no matter what is going on in your life. Whenever you see a fun run event and all the spectators cheering from the sidelines, you know that the encouragement from the cheerleaders on the sidelines has kept many of those runners moving toward the finish line. The cheering has motivated them to continue to the finish line. Consumers seek out motivation as much as anything else when they make a buying decision. If people know that there will be a healthy dose of motivation at the fitness club to keep them coming back, they are happier and more satisfied with their decision to exercise. When people join a gym, they know they will be motivated either by the facility, the staff, or others who are working out at the same time. When it comes to exercising, there is nothing better than meeting up with gym buddies in the weight room or the aerobics studio.

Doctor's Orders—An increasing number of people are being told by their doctors to go to a gym. I remember a client who had a prescription with her, signed by her doctor, that read: *Join a gym.* She had walked into a drug store and presented the piece of paper to the pharmacist who promptly told her that she was in the wrong place. This woman was so completely programmed to simply take a pill that she was in shock when she realized that she had not even read the prescription before hitting the pharmacy. We sold a membership to that woman, and to many others who were under "doctor's orders" to exercise. What was so interesting about this was the fact that this woman would not have been able to begin an exercise regime if simply *told* to do so; she required a *prescription.* More and more doctors are understanding that if they recommend exercise to a patient, the patients are more likely to comply if they are supported in an exercise program.

Happiness—In our culture, *happiness* is recognized as not only a possibility, but also a common goal, and this concept is frequently discussed in the news, popular magazines, and other forms of media. Many people feel that joining a gym and exercising is a way of being happier. Being a personal trainer requires conducting very thorough assessments of potential clients. The most frequent theme that emerges as people disclose their feelings around exercise and what motivates them is that of improved happiness and enjoyment of life. They may not always state it directly, but it is almost always part of their intent in pursuing fitness goals. Happiness seems elusive when we are in physical pain, don't feel good in our skin, or have health issues that limit our enjoyment of life. Joining a gym and exercising is generally perceived as a step toward being in a happier state in one's life.

Whatever one's reasons for joining a gym, the one thing that can be guaranteed is that it is a great decision. At this time, fewer than twenty percent of Canadian adults belong to a fitness facility. This needs to change in order to improve the health of individual people as well as the health of our nation. Fitness is prevention, and prevention is the best cure.

All levels of government are affected by rising health care costs. We all have a responsibility to ourselves and our families to take care of our health just as we take care of our finances. My experience as a gym owner reinforced my belief in the value of fitness centers and their role in creating a healthier community. After my business sold, I decided to commit to paper my heart's strongest desire – which is to be a part of a positive change and the human potential movement – and write this book that you now hold in your hands. Everyone has the potential to be and do what they desire. It is difficult to focus on our purpose when we are in pain, out of shape, tired or suffering from debilitating health issues. Joining a gym and focusing on exercise is a way to gain the ability to do the things that you really, really want to do. We told our clients daily that they did not have to love exercise, but they had to love their life enough to exercise in order to get the most out of living.

I hope that as you read this book and understand intellectually and emotionally the value of your health, that you embrace your wild side. Let your dreams become a reality and don't hold back. If you want to ride your bike across the country, do it. If you want to go into Tough Mudder, do it. If you want to be super fit and compete as an athlete until your last dying breath, do it. Don't let the judgments of others or your own inner critic alter your fitness goals and dreams. You will read stories about some extraordinary people in this book and read stats about probabilities if you don't claim your right to a healthy body and mind. Choose to let your "exercise freak fly" and let it take you on grand adventures. Embrace any possibility that the mind can imagine. Remember that this life is not a dress rehearsal so grab the best costume you can find and take your place on stage and act out the life you have been dreaming of. My gift to you is my words and my unconditional support while you enter into this new way of being.

My dream is that once fifty percent or more of the population is going to a gym regularly to exercise, a whole new world will be opened up to everyone. There will be more money for education and poverty prevention as fewer funds are needed for health care. New and ingenious methods of exercise will be invented. Gym facilities will be designed in interesting and creative ways to focus on the needs of a wide variety of consumers. As people become fitter and healthier, communication will improve and there will be less violence and misery. Energy will be available for community enhancing projects that bring people together in a positive way. There really is no end to the possibilities for improving the quality of life through increased health and fitness. Gyms are at the forefront of this change. As a gym owner, I found it difficult to explain the value of quality fitness facilities in a community without seeming self-serving. Now I have the freedom to express that value in a book and explore new ways to be a part of creating a positive change in the world.

I wrote this book to inspire those of you making the choice to be healthier to get to a gym and start that journey. Included in the book are tips on how to choose a gym and how to manage the first few weeks and months of your gym experience. There are chapters on the basics of exercise physiology to help explain why your body needs regular exercise, and chapters on saving your brain, as well as some different perspectives on health and wellness. This book can be read straight through or used as a reference when questions come up.

As I was starting to write this book, I joined a writer's group at the local library. I sat next to a gentleman who was composing a memoir on his journey with cancer. He politely asked me what I was writing about. "I am writing a book on joining a gym," I responded. Without hesitation, he immediately said, "I need to join a gym." My desire is that many more people will have a similar reaction and head out to the "club" and sign the papers: the first step in living a happier, healthier, and more engaged life.

Wishing you all the success in your journey of health and fitness.

Sheena Bull, 2014

1:
Eight Common Misconceptions About the Gym

Strong relationships are one of life's great joys, and building one from the ground up can feel like a significant accomplishment. In order to build any kind of relationship, it is important to clear up any misconceptions that will eventually come up in a conversation. Some of these conversations may include confessions like "Actually, I am not a good cook," or "Just to let you know, I hate foreign films with subtitles," or "My idea of camping is checking into a five-star resort. Just saying!" Relationships quickly become strained when there are expectations that are not met. When it comes to your gym, it is essential from the very beginning to know your expectations in order to ensure a long-term and rewarding relationship. In order for these expectations to take shape, there are some misconceptions about fitness facilities that need to be cleared up. Here are eight of the most common misconceptions, and the reasons we need to start thinking differently about the gym.

GYMS ARE FOR YOUNG PEOPLE

Exercise becomes increasingly important as we get older. In fact, the amount of exercise we require is directly proportional to our age. For example, if a twenty-year-old requires twenty minutes of exercise per day, then a 70-year-old needs 70 minutes of exercise per day. (There are many reasons for this – such as the fact that as we age we tend to naturally slow down as physical demands diminish on the job and at home– and these are covered in detail later in this book). Fitness facilities recognize this and are including programs for all age groups.

Unfortunately, most of the marketing used by gyms has focused on young, fit bodies. This causes problems in terms of our perceptions of fitness facilities. When it comes to making a decision about whether to join a gym, it is easy to talk yourself out of it if you believe it is really only a place for young people. A gym is for everybody and is much more diverse and dynamic when a range of age groups participate. At my former gym, we had a 92-year-old woman who worked with a trainer every week. *Everyone* loved her, especially the younger women. Her dedication inspired them, and they came to see that they, too, could be vital and energetic right into their nineties.

As our society becomes more aware of the need for action toward better health, we can only hope that the marketing and advertising for gyms become more authentic, relevant, and inclusive. As the population ages, there will be an increase in the average age of people choosing to join fitness clubs, which is hopeful and inspiring. Just remember that if your gym does seem to have relatively youthful members, and you are in an older category, the mixing of generations makes for a vibrant, motivational atmosphere.

GYMS ARE TOO EXPENSIVE

This is all too often a belief that prevents people from joining a fitness facility. There are many different types of gyms, especially in larger cities, and membership costs vary depending on the type of gym and the location. If you are on a tight budget, the monthly cost can be a factor. Membership costs usually increase when extras are included in the package. Some pricey clubs have extras such as pools, hot tubs, and a complimentary towel service while bare-bones gyms are more affordable. The average price for a gym membership in North America is around 50 dollars per month. There are clubs that are twenty dollars a month and clubs that are over 100 dollars a month. While this may seem like an unrealistic or frivolous expense, keep in mind that it is an investment in your future. It can also be extremely costly to be sick, injured, or have long term medical issues related to lack of physical fitness.

One of the reasons that people believe gym memberships are too expensive is that many individuals purchase memberships and then stop going to the gym. When one buys a product and never uses that product, it is easy to feel that money was spent and nothing was gained. The reality, however, is that the *gym* was there the whole time providing all the services promised when the membership documents were signed. It was the *membership* that was not used. Though the financial commitment motivates many people to go to the gym, many stop going because their pocketbooks were not affected *enough*. Ironically, if gym memberships were more expensive, perhaps, members would be motivated to go more often.

In the meantime, I can assure you that gyms have never been more affordable. Here's a free tip for you: when you commit to buying your membership, make sure you use it and enjoy the feeling of receiving tremendous value for the money you spent.

JOINING A GYM MEANS LOSING WEIGHT

This is a big one as countless times over the years I have heard people lamenting that they joined a gym but did not lose a pound. This common complaint makes it sound as if joining a gym were synonymous to weight loss. It was a red flag to me if a new member joined my gym with the sole purpose of losing weight. (For more details about the issues surrounding weight loss, read on).

If weight loss is the primary goal when joining a gym, and the goal is not achieved, people often perceive the gym to be at fault. This type of reasoning is, of course, illogical and would be enough to cause those who use reason, like Spock from Star Trek, to break out in hives. Yet, it is common and generates misunderstanding. During our staff training sessions, we were all clear that we did not want our club marketed as a place to lose weight. Instead, we viewed our gym as a vehicle to engage in a healthy lifestyle. As far as I am concerned, the issue of weight loss and attending a gym are two separate concepts. When contemplating a life change, framing it in a positive way helps create the change we desire. It is easy to say "I am joining a gym to begin a proactive approach to living a healthy life." That message is very differ-ent from saying, "I am joining the gym for three months to lose these extra ten pounds I seem to have put on."

Success in life can never be measured by how many pounds are lost through dieting or exercising. True success is how we treat our bodies and others in our lives. Joining a gym means that you respect your body enough to look after it. Kudos to you!

GYMS ARE FOR FIT PEOPLE

What? Do we take trousers to the tailor to be hemmed if they're already the perfect length? I don't think so. Gyms are a place where people who are not fit become fit. Plus, gyms are for everybody. It is true that gyms attract really fit people because these individuals have a passion for fitness and love to be in a supportive environment, but gyms are actually meant to maintain an environment that attracts those who do not like to exercise. It seems that only a small percentage of the population has a personality that loves fitness while the other 90 percent is not so in love with fitness. If you are not excited about working out, then hitting the gym can be a perfect solution. Once you are there, you feel motivated by the energetic environment and by others who are exercising. At the club, you do not have the option to engage in activi-ties that are not exercise related. In addition, as you become fitter, you will have compassion for your friends and family members who feel intimidated by the process of exercise and use your experience to help them along the right path. Share your experience with them and it may inspire the people in your circle of influence to try out the gym.

YOU NEED TO GO TO THE GYM EVERY DAY

This belief almost certainly will create a tragic ending. Trying to get to the gym every day, especially if you are new to exercise or "de-conditioned," which is an inclusive way of saying out of shape, is not realistic. This is the number one reason people don't keep their new year's resolutions.

The amount of exercise to maintain general health is different than the amount needed to improve your fitness level. The recommended amount of exercise is 150 minutes of moderate-intensity exercise per week for health benefits. Exercising any more than that moves you into the arena of becoming fitter. When a newbie to the gym walked through our doors, I always told them that, in the beginning, less is more. First of all, trying to make a lifestyle change requires energy. It is best to use less energy when starting out or both your body and your brain will resist the new challenge. If you can hit the gym once a week, you are still helping your body. When you begin to feel more relaxed about going to the gym, try making it twice a week or adding an aerobics class to make it three times. Remember that this is a lifetime commitment. Like any other relationship, starting slowly and getting comfortable is always recommended.

YOU HAVE TO LIKE TO EXERCISE TO JOIN A GYM

When you see all those pictures of happy people exercising, it can seem that everybody who engages in fitness loves it. This couldn't be further from the truth. Remember that 90 percent of the population is not enthusiastic about working up a sweat. This is the very reason that programs like Zumba took off at lightning speed. Zumba, a dance program where the goal is fun and exercise is a by-product, was created to be geared towards the 90 percent who don't love exercise (If you have not tried Zumba, make sure you do!) And if it turns out dance isn't your bag, there are plenty of other group fitness programs that have been put together to bring fun to fitness.

Despite the fact that most people are not raving fans of exercise, they still have a desire to be healthy and fit. If you like to be motivated, have fun, find a sense of community, engage in healthy activities, feel energetic, or are under doctor's orders, – it sounds like you've got more than enough reason to head to the gym. You don't have to love to exercise, but you will love the results, and that is what will keep you going back.

YOU HAVE TO BE HEALTHY TO JOIN A GYM

Over the years, many people have expressed to me their need to get fit or healthy *before* getting a gym membership. I tell them that the gym is the place to go if they have an injury or an illness where exercise is not contraindicated. The gym is the place to *get healthy*. That said, it is essential to discuss this with your doctor and to be cleared to start an exercise program. If you are in the acute phase of your injury, medical attention and physiotherapy is the way to go. However, once the visits to the physiotherapist end, it is essential to start a proper exercise routine, both to avoid a long-term chronic condition and to keep the rest of your body functioning properly.

If you have a degenerative condition like high cholesterol, high blood pressure, adult onset diabetes, or arthritis, it is critical to engage in a regular exercise program. Your exercise program may require modifications, but when it comes to getting healthy, being sedentary is not an option. In fact, the positive psychological effects of being in an upbeat, energetic atmosphere are enormous. In an ideal world, everyone would exercise regularly *before* suffering from an accident or medical condition, but not being in perfect health is no excuse for avoiding the gym. There are numerous scientific studies that prove the benefits of exercise even after a medical event like a heart attack. The AHA (American Heart Association) has released 'Scientific Statements' to this effect: http://circ.aha-journals.org/content/107/24/3109.full.

I know that many of us like to clean up the house before the housekeeper shows up, but our health is a totally different matter. There is no guarantee that exercise will improve your health, but it is guaranteed that remaining sedentary will make your condition worse.

ALL GYMS ARE THE SAME

Gyms come in all shapes and sizes. For the purpose of this book, I would consider a gym to be any facility that provides its members access to exercise. There are massive facilities, like the Calgary Winter Club, that have everything from a weight room to hockey rinks, to full-service restaurants. Then there are small gyms, like Snap 24-hour fitness franchises, which exist in smaller communities and are open 24 hours to members, but only staffed for a few hours a day. Ten years ago, the women-only Curves franchise was one of the fastest growing franchises in North America and are still well attended. At a typical Curves, you will find very minimal equipment, but the atmosphere is fun and the routine is short. Then, of course, there are the large gym chains such as Goodlife Fitness. Both the large chain clubs and the independent standalone facilities have benefits. The important thing to keep in mind is what you are looking for as the consumer, and what is available in an area that suits you. Some people are only interested in yoga classes, so they choose a yoga studio that does not have a weight room. Others are looking for a wide variety of weight equipment and are not interested in an aerobics studio. There are those who prefer a community recreation center that has a pool and hot tub attached to the workout area. If you have a long commute to work, a fitness center closer to work for the noon hour workout may be the best option. If you're a shift worker, you probably need a facility that allows access after normal business hours. It is essential to make a list of your needs and make your choice dependent on the gym meeting those requirements.

No matter what your final decision is, it is not set in stone and you have the freedom to change gyms if you so choose. Just be sure to use the gym regularly and develop a relationship with the staff and other members. Feel free to become part of the gym's community and get involved, stay on track, make suggestions if you have any, and above all, have fun!

2:

The Best Exercise Program is the One You're Doing

Personal trainers are frequently asked, "What is the best exercise program?" As a new trainer, I was faced with this constant inquiry, and in response, I would launch into my usual monolog, unleashing a complicated and exhaustive explanation upon the unlucky soul who ventured to ask the question. Then one day, after a few years of working as a trainer and trying to overlook the glazed-over expressions and barely suppressed yawns of gym-goers, I had an "Aha!" moment.

When I had this small epiphany, even though I had previously bored my clients with my monolog, my brain took a turn out of a well-worn rut and I decided to be clear and direct with them. It may have been confidence or maybe it was experience or maybe a combination of the two, but it was a moment within a moment that is forever memorable. It changed the way I interacted with clients about their exercise program.

On the day of the epiphany, a client arrived at the studio with a book under her arm. She was a new client and was very curious about her program. She always double checked my advice and guidance. Every session she brought a newspaper clipping or a magazine that suggested various ways to exercise, wanting to pick apart the articles like a monkey combing through another family member's hair looking for bugs. But the problem was that this woman, as with many of my other clients, was never actually stuck to a routine long enough to see good results.

Finally, as my client pulled out her book and began to show me pages that were dog-eared and full of bookmarks, my mind took a sudden turn. Instead of just politely nodding and patiently listening, I found myself saying, "Actually, the best exercise program is the one that you are doing." The words escaped my mouth like a slippery fish getting away before I even thought about what I was saying. The moment had finally arrived for me to take charge and set my client straight. This comment quickly became one of my favorite sayings and is still the best way to express the bottom line to people who fuss and argue about the latest research or trendy exercise fad.

No matter how great your exercise program is, how many books are written about it, how many TV shows or YouTube videos are watched, *if you are not participating in it*, clearly, it is not the best. This statement gets people's attention and brings them back to reality.

Often, we are so busy thinking, reading, and questioning what is the best for us, that we forget to actually do what we need to do. The takeaway message from reading this book is that if you start an exercise program and it's not working, do something else. This is not like a career, having a baby, or getting a puppy. You are not tied to any specific program, gym, or group. One beautiful aspect of the fitness industry is the flexibility and choice that is offered. There is no one-size-fits-all in fitness. Everyone is an individual with their own body type, gender, age, lifestyle, goals, and dreams. At the same time, however, all the different possible exercise programs and facilities can be confounding to newcomers and those who have been on an exercise sabbatical. While the best program is the one you are doing, first you must start by finding the one that you're most likely to start and keep doing. This chapter provides some examples of different types of programs that are available, and who they may best suit, as well as some suggestions for activities that can be combined to create your own individual strategy for the "best" results.

What is Exercise?

First of all, I need to be clear about what is and what isn't exercise. To qualify an aerobics program as exercise, you need to gain the results of health and fitness. For health and fitness results, your heart rate needs to be increased to at least 60 percent of your maximal heart rate (MHR) and kept up for over thirty minutes. (MHR can be estimated by the mathematical equation 220 minus your age.)

In terms of weight resistant exercises, you need to be adding more resistance or including exercises for all major muscle groups regularly to consider this program a benefit to your overall health and fitness.

WHAT IS NOT EXERCISE

It is easy to give the *appearance* of exercising while not actually reaping the benefits of exercising. While the activities may be enjoyable, in doing the activity, you will not reap the same excellent benefits of exercise.

Golfing is not exercise, especially if you use a cart to travel the course. It can be a great social activity and, while the walking component is active, generally we can't consider it exercise, especially if the game ends with a beer and French fries.

Gardening is not always exercise. I am prepared to go out on a limb here, with the possibility of the branch breaking. My years of experience with clients is that when they say that they are exercising through gardening, it is impossible to qualify the type of activity, the intensity, the duration and the frequency at which they are exercising. On Salt Spring Island, the biggest club, by far, is the gardening club. As a result, many gardeners would join the gym and list gardening as their exercise program. When asked detailed questions, the member would agree that watering plants is not really exercise and sitting on a stool to weed the garden cannot be considered exercise either, but they could point out various injuries that were a result of some of the heavier chores attempted in gardening when they were not fit enough. In fact, the garden season only lasts for six months at the most, leaving even the most avid gardeners inactive for a good portion of the year. Because of the many variables in the whole arena of gardening, like golf, it is active, but not to be listed as a strategy for specific health benefits.

Sitting on a recumbent bike at the gym and reading is not exercise, but it is a great way to warm up. It is more active than just sitting while reading, but if you can focus your eyes on your copy of *Golfer's Digest* while on the bike, you are definitely not focused on increasing your breathing.

Restorative yoga is not exercise, but it is relaxing and a lovely activity for meditation and breathing. As a matter of fact, many stretch classes are not exercise. There are benefits to your body when you stretch and practice breathing such as feeling and awareness of your body, but exercise has to involve achieving physiological changes to your body through increased aerobic capacity and muscular strength. My first-ever yoga class was instructed by a seventy-year-old yoga master who had studied and taught Iyengar yoga for 40 years. I recall that it was a great experience, and after the class, the instructor expressed her surprise at how well I took to the program, considering that I was new to yoga. It occurred to me as I looked around at the other participants, that they would actually get more out of the class if they were to lift weights and do a cardio program in addition to yoga; both activities that I engage in regularly. Balancing on one leg while holding your body still requires strength and stamina, which can only be developed through yoga with time. Don't forget that yoga gurus practice for hours a day. We are fortunate to have other options in terms of exercise equipment in order to maintain our fitness levels with significantly less of a time commitment than was historically required for a serious yoga practice.

The best thing you can do to take the confusion out of exercise is to keep a journal to track how much exercise you are getting on a weekly and monthly basis. The goal is to aim for six hours of exercise, *on average per week*, over a period of a year. It is best to add up your hours over a month and divide by four to get an average per week for the month. The goal is not to get all 24 hours of exercise in one week, as it is best if it is spread out over the month. Having said that, looking at the big picture instead of a snapshot will be more accurate and helpful for exercise adherence. Recording and monitoring your physical activities is very motivating, and being able to review results of an entire month gives a much more accurate representation of your progress than a daily or weekly total.

Let's take a look at a one-month period of time for two different individuals, Dave, and Molly. Dave is very athletic and maintains a high level of fitness, and Molly is interested in just staying healthy and fit. Dave plays ice hockey twice a week for an hour at a time and also hits the gym for two, hour-long sessions a week to lift weights. That's about all the time he has for exercise since he has a full-time job and a young family. Nonetheless, he also regularly takes his children hiking and walking, carrying the youngest on his back. This also amounts to about two hours a week, which means Dave accumulates an average of six hours of exercise per week.

Molly, on the other hand, likes to get out for a walk/run with her friends three times a week for 90 minutes a session. She also goes to a power yoga class once a week at her gym. Molly sees a personal trainer twice a week to lift weights and tries to get to the gym at least once a week on her own. Because she has a full-time desk job, Molly makes an effort to stop sitting once she finishes work. As a result of this lifestyle choice, Molly chooses to be without a car and live only a few blocks from work so she can walk to work. Her children have moved to other cities so she now lives alone, but she has many friends within walking distance whom she visits. Altogether, Molly accumulates almost nine hours a week of exercise.

Dave's monthly total is 24 hours, but when translated into the longer term, things look a bit different: in the spring and summer, Dave goes out road bike riding with his friends for about six hours a week. That brings his total exercise hours up to 48 per month for six months of the year. Molly accumulates 36 hours of exercise per month regularly, but in the warmer months, she hikes with friends on weekends for four to six hours at a time, adding twenty extra hours to the spring and summer months. Her monthly hours of exercise are bumped up to 56 hours for six months of the year.

This method of counting hours of exercise does not take into account the intensity of the exercise as that is difficult to recommend in a book and without a proper face to face conversation. It depends on an individual's age, health status, and willingness to exert themselves intensely. I encourage my clients to count any activity that gets their heart rate up or causes muscle fatigue and is done for the purpose of being active. When you look at both David and Molly, you can see how quickly they accumulate hours of exercise. If they miss a week, it does not affect the overall numbers. It is important to think in big chunks of time because if you focus on missing a day or even a few days, you can lose sight of the big picture and quickly become discouraged. Make sure you keep track of all your exercise hours and feel the satisfaction when you notice the hours going up in a given month and of the accomplishments that result from that effort.

Notice that both Molly and Dave balance their exercise program between the gym and the outdoors. This is smart because having a wide range of activities keeps you interested and motivated. While going for a bike ride or a hike in the sunshine with friends and family may seem like the ideal exercise to many people, it is essential to have an indoor space to use during bad weather. That is why it is important to have access to a gym or studio during those times when being outside is not practical, and in some places that could be up to eight months of the year.

The gym will also have a wide variety of programs to choose from to keep you motivated, committed, and challenged. For example, resistance exercises can be done as part of a circuit class if that motivates you more than lifting weights on your own. Curves built a whole business by focusing on exercising in a circuit that women can get into or leave whenever they want and deliberately design a shorter program that suits many women. If you are taking regular yoga classes, not restorative yoga, count the hours for them in your weekly exercise total. There are some very intense yoga classes available, and they can be an interesting change from a regular, routine program. There is various boot camp–style classes both indoors and outdoors. Cross-Fit is a brand of boot camp style exercise that has become popular over the last few years, leading to many fitness studios being solely Cross-Fit gyms.

Plan an Exercise Program

TRX

When planning activities to involve in our exercise programs, we can't forget martial arts classes like judo and karate. There has also been a new trend toward spin classes, which are offered both at full-service gyms and spin only studios. The TRX is still a great way to train both solo and in a class format. If you are unfamiliar with the TRX system, it is an exercise program originally developed by the Army for soldiers to maintain fitness when equipment is not available. The TRX straps have handles and clips to change the length of the straps. The straps are designed to be placed in a doorway or around a post. They are light weight and many athletes take them in their suitcase while they are on the road. There are studios with hooks in the ceiling for the TRX straps, allowing entire classes of people to train together. It is worth taking the time to look at the TRX website for an idea of the exercises and versatility of this simple but effective piece of equipment.

AEROBICS

There are still the traditional step aerobics classes as well as a new generation of aerobics including Zumba, Bellyfit, and NIA (Non-Impact Aerobics). These classes are dance-focused and are fun as well as challenging.

PILATES OR YOGA

Another popular practice is Pilates, which ranges in techniques from using beds called reformers and other props, to simple mat exercises. There are private Pilates studios as well as Pilates classes offered as part of a full aerobics studio. Many people prefer private one-on-one instruction rather than group classes. Those who are new to an exercise method, like Pilates, often find it beneficial to have personal instruction before joining a group. Having individual attention creates confidence and, ultimately, better results, with less opportunity for injury.

This is just to name a few different types of exercise to get you started on the road to finding the right combination of activities to create a complete program that works best for you. The purpose here has been to let you know how many choices you have and how to look at the big picture. Not all exercise has to be intense. It depends on the goals of the exercise itself and the goals of the participant. Whatever you decide to try out and participate in, please be sure to make note of it in your exercise journal. If you find your weekly and monthly totals increasing, you probably have found the exercise program that works for you. If your totals start to decline, it may be time to try something new or rearrange your schedule if it's a challenge to find the time for the exercise. The important message is that the best exercise program is the one that you are doing. If someone tells you about the latest and greatest exercise fad do not feel discouraged if you have not jumped on the bandwagon. If you are doing what you enjoy and doing it routinely with enthusiasm, you are participating in the very best program there is.

3:

The Secret Weapon of Celebrities

Not long ago, my friend Lori invited me to have dinner at her house. When I arrived, her TV was on and she was watching a news program about the Hollywood workout scene. "Sheena, you should watch this," she said and gestured toward the couch for me to sit down. After a few minutes of watching the show, I turned to her and said, "What message are you taking away from this news report?" Lori did not miss a beat as she responded, "That even movie stars need a personal trainer." "Good answer," I said, smiling at my buddy.

My friendship with Lori began the day she drove up to my building in her hot little, green, convertible Audi. She was looking for the computer business that had previously occupied space in the commercial building that was home to my gym. I happened to be in the space with a client at the time and noticed this attractive redhead trying to open the front door. I walked over and opened the door and asked this bewildered woman if I could help her. When I found out why she was there, I told her that the computer store had closed shop. When I told her it was now a gym, her immediate response was, "I need to go to a gym. I *really* need to go to a gym." Lori looked frustrated at not finding the computer store. "I was hoping to get my computer fixed," she said as stood in the room assuming the annoyed posture. Then she grinned and held out her arms and said, "But you know summer is coming and I dread the idea of short sleeve tops." She waved her right arm, jiggling the flab with her left hand. "Look at you," she laughed. "You probably have never jiggled anywhere, ever." Then the typical rant began. "I, on the other hand, hate the flab on the back of my arms, my stomach is getting out of control, not to mention my skinny legs. But I can't seem to get motivated. I just keep obsessing over all these problem areas."

"Well then," I said. "I happen to have solutions for your concerns." After a 30-minute tour of the gym and a chat about her needs with regards to an exercise program, Lori walked away with a one-year membership and a personal training package. This started a two-year long relationship that consisted of exercise and friendship. Now, when we hang out, Lori and I will occasionally share a laugh about how much the trip to the non-existent computer store cost her: an increase in her line of credit, litres of sweat, and years of sore muscles.

Personal Training is Changing World Health, One Body at a Time!

Lori quickly understood the benefits of having a trainer, because, without that extra push, her self-motivation was limited. There has to be someone to hold you accountable when you are engaged in an exercise program. Trust me, it is not a good idea to be accountable to a spouse or other family member. The easiest way to strain a relationship is to nag your significant other about hitting the gym. Instead, try offering a gift of personal training sessions, then leave it up to the trainer to be the enforcer. (You will thank me later for this advice.)

During the TV program that Lori and I watched about the fitness scene in LA, that need for accountability was reinforced. The reporter mentioned that a certain personal trainer in Hollywood had a five-year waiting list. He may be more popular than the Dalai Lama. (Hard to believe? This is LA we're talking about!) The cameras showed clips of gyms that were built underground, complete with special security systems and personal trainers who had to sign waivers to guarantee the privacy and safety of their clients. They mentioned some of the most famous actors in Hollywood and gave a list of their trainers and exercise programs.

In spite of the fact that these actors' bodies are their ticket to fame and fortune, and that without the right look they would never even make it to an audition, let alone get a gig, most cannot work out successfully unless they have a trainer. My friend Lori understands this and knows that you need more than motivation. She knows you need an appointment. Her career may not depend on her fitness level, but her enjoyment of life certainly does. The next time you feel guilty about needing a personal trainer, or read somewhere that trainers are an unnecessary expense or that gyms are just trying to sell you on another product, remember all those celebrities working out in LA. Even though they risk losing their career and lifestyle without that fit, healthy look, most celebrities, and other successful individuals find it difficult to exercise without a personal trainer. So when you finally bite the bullet and commit to an exercise program with a trainer, remember that you have discovered the secret weapon of these famous actors. Hiring a trainer to help you only means that you are a proactive individual who is clever enough to invest in your health.

My career as a personal trainer has been a rewarding one. Over the years, I have had the privilege of mentoring new trainers and watching them also fall in love with the profession as they became confident, educated, and inspired. While working in the fitness business is rewarding, being a trainer is also a calling. Not everyone lasts as a trainer, but everyone who tries it is forever changed. I often think that personal trainers, in their own way, are on the front lines of life, helping their clients find health and fitness in a world that supports the opposite. Brené Brown, the motivational speaker and author of *Daring Greatly* (2012), says it clearly when she states that we are the most in-debt, obese, addicted, and medicated adult cohort in the history of North America. Every day, personal trainers are in the trenches, coaching, nagging, motivating, and appealing to their clients to get out and stay out of that unhealthy majority. As trainers, we need to be impeccable with our own health habits. If we have worked eight consecutive hours, it can be hard to be motivated to hit the treadmill for that 30-minute run. We get tired, burnt out, and frustrated just like everyone else, but what keeps us going are the positive changes we see take place every day. Seeing and feeling the difference that our work is making in the lives of our clients and their families motivates us. It's like throwing a stone into the water and watching the ripples move outward. The stone, like changes to a body, may be small but the ripple effect is enormous.

FIVE REASONS TO USE A PERSONAL TRAINER

1. You will show up for an appointment.
2. You will see better results up to three times faster.
3. You will avoid injuring yourself.
4. You will not get bored.
5. You will have the support and encouragement you need to get over exercise humps.

PERSONAL TRAINERS HAVE THEIR OWN STYLE

As with any profession, there are many types of personal trainers, each with their own expertise related to different aspects of fitness. As a consumer, it is essential to investigate personal trainers before hiring one. Find out who they are and what they charge before making a final decision on the best fit for you. If you are new to exercise and feel intimidated by the process, an experienced trainer who is perhaps less edgy and more gentle may be an appropriate choice.

If, however, you are training for a Tough Mudder event or a powerlifting competition, you may want a trainer who is extroverted and maybe even a bit pushy. The age of the trainer and his or her fitness level become less important as you develop a relationship and recognize that *looks* don't always correlate to *skill* when it comes to being an impact-ful trainer. It is important to feel comfortable and connected with the trainer you are considering. Whether or not a connection exists will be obvious within the first few minutes of the meeting.

While you are out shopping for a gym that meets your criteria, research the personal training department. If the personal trainers are independent contractors, they will not be under the supervision of a gym manager, and therefore, the process of hiring a trainer will require more rigorous screening on your part.

In my experience, a personal trainer who works on their own, under their own supervision, doesn't always have the advantage of mentorship and feedback, which are two areas that serve to promote their improvement. Personally, I am a fan of clubs that hire their trainers as employees. Not only are they under supervision, which gives them the benefit of consistent development, but clients can also rotate through several different trainers. Additionally, if the trainers are on staff, the manager can be involved in matching the right trainer with the right client. One sure way to stop your body from adapting to exercise is to switch to a new trainer who may bring a different set of skills. Many of my clients were amazed at how a different trainer could change the way their body responded to the same exercises.

Another problem with always working with only one trainer is accommodating time off for both the personal trainer and the client, which is necessary both for holidays and as a break in routine. Clients who become attached to one particular trainer can make it difficult for their favorite trainer to get away. Likewise, when the client goes on holiday it can cause a significant drop in the trainer's income if they are unable to find a replacement client.

Before you have a trial run at a gym, be sure to ask about the training staff, and also thoroughly check out the gym's website to find out more about their trainers. While doing your research, you may notice a personal trainer on the website that you think will be a good fit. Feel free to request a complimentary session with that trainer. Before booking, make sure that the trainer you are considering has a current certification. Certified trainers have access to liability insurance and have gone through a rigorous certification process, holding them more accountable to maintain industry standards. Remember this is your body! Be bold and ask for what you want and be clear about need.

CONSIDER YOUR TIME AND BUDGET WHEN CHOOSING A PERSONAL TRAINER

Then there are the questions of budget and time, both of which bring varying constraints into the equation for many people who train. There is nothing wrong with hiring a junior trainer if it means you can get more sessions for the same amount you would spend on a senior trainer. New trainers have tremendous energy and enthusiasm. In addition, new trainers need a chance to practice their skills. Of course, the experience of a skilled, knowledgeable trainer is not to be dismissed, especially for those with injuries or those looking for sport-specific training. When it comes to scheduling, the first thing you have to decide is how many times a week you will need a trainer. Three times a week is ideal, but that is not possible for everyone. While you're getting yourself set up on a new program, I suggest seeing a trainer once a week, followed up by a second weekly session on your own. After a few months of this, clients quite often find that they begin seeing a trainer twice a week, mainly because they need that second appointment to get them back into the gym.

Other clients discover that they are fine to work out on their own and prefer not to be bound by an appointment. These independent individuals often prefer a twice-per-month or once-per-month session with their trainer. In any case, making those appointments, even just once a month, keeps members coming back to the gym. And this, as we know, is the key because the best exercise program is the one you are doing!

WHAT WILL YOUR PERSONAL TRAINING SESSION BE LIKE?

It would be perfectly understandable if, at this point, you found yourself wondering, "What exactly does a personal trainer *do*?" Lori, who had never worked with a personal trainer, wondered the same thing when she arrived for her first training session. She was nervous. She was anxious about her abilities, my expectations, and the potential soreness her body could incur. Trainers take their time getting to know their clients before increasing the difficulty of the program. Lori was new to training and the gym, and as a result, it took a few sessions just to get used to the gym equipment. As Lori became used to the gym and the exercises, I paid attention to her posture and the muscles that were weak. As it turns out, Lori had a few postural issues and weak muscles, but not a weak spirit. In fact, Lori wore a t-shirt to her first session that said "Member of the National Sarcasm Society…like we need your support," and I knew immediately that she was going to be a great client. We worked on strengthening her weak muscles, by gradually increasing the weights. We mobilized her back with the foam roller and worked on the core with balance exercises and body ball exercises. She would sweat, swear and then thank me for a great time. She grinned in delight at how great she felt and how well her clothes fit her.

Depending on your fitness level and gym experience, a trainer can either take full responsibility for each one of your workouts or design a program that you do on your own, meeting with you several times a month. The two methods seem to be used equally with the general population, but it takes about six months to know where you are the most comfortable. Finding a personal trainer is an individual decision. Take the time to decide and, as mentioned above, give consideration to your budget and what kind of exerciser you are.

Sometimes it happens that a client realizes their personal trainer is not a good fit for them. If this happens to you, don't avoid your workouts. Your trainer will not take it personally if you decide to change trainers. Trainers are professionals and know better than anyone how important the dynamics between trainer and client are. Go and see the gym manager and ask for their assistance in finding someone else. Remember, their top priority and yours is to keep you happy and keep you exercising.

PERSONAL TRAINERS ARE NOT JUST FOR CELEBRITIES

Celebrities have known about the secret weapon of personal trainers for years. At one time, only the wealthy could afford to hire a trainer, but luckily, this luxury has become much more affordable over the last twenty years. Personal training is no longer considered a luxury, but a necessity by many people. My friend Lori found out that having a trainer really works, and that it is one of the best investments you can make for your health. During our sessions, Lori would tell me about hearing her colleagues talk about their gym memberships that they never used. They talked about diets and cleanses that they couldn't stick with and about aches and pains that they considered part of aging. They also discussed the constant stream of goodies and treats that no one needed, constantly appearing in the office. It reaffirmed to her that a personal trainer is the commitment that everyone needs, not only to be motivated to show up to the session, but to visualize the trainer asking for 20 more push-ups and 20 more lunges followed by 20 more reverse crunches, every time a cookie sits on a plate in the office, every time the lazy-boy looks oh-so-comfortable, and every time that bag of excuses floats around in the mind like a watch hypnotizing the person staring at it. When you have a trainer, immediately thoughts of the future training session snap the wandering, undisciplined mind back to a new and better reality. This new reality is working out with a trainer to get rid of aches and pains, tighten ab muscles, and gain increased energy and renewed zest for life.

My clients, including Lori, red-faced and sweating, would often say to me during their sessions, "... And to think that

I pay for this torture!" I did what needed to be done to help them reach their health goals.

During your training sessions, don't be afraid to have fun. Trainers need a little ribbing every once in a while. Be difficult and let your inner 'bitch' out sometimes. It will make the session end sooner and help you release all that pent up energy. Do whatever you need to do in order to get results and keep going back for more. By more, I mean more fun, better results, and the satisfaction of being proactive instead of complaining. Lori still has her wit and makes me laugh, but she feels the positive vibe of taking charge and doing something to stop the not so great changes that will occur if one is sedentary. Sometimes she wears the 'Sarcasm Society' t-shirt and sometimes she wears the 'I am Heavily Medicated for your Protection' tank top to her workouts. Lori may not have perfect arms, but she has a perfect sense of humor and keeps coming back for the *more* that a personal trainer and gym membership offer her.

4:
Let's Get Started

The first step to your new, fit life is locating all the gyms that are close to your home or workplace. Everyone likes convenience, which is a reason people profess to be more satisfied with their gym. – People claim on surveys to like their gym if it has a convenient location. Plus, exercise adherence depends on an easily accessible fitness center. Once you have created a shortlist, it's time to physically check out each potential club.

Choosing a Gym

Ask for a complimentary walk-through at any facility that you are considering. The type of equipment is the most important feature. A pool, sauna, and hot tub are lovely extras, but if the equipment is outdated or lacking in any way, it may not be the best choice for a great workout.

CHECK OUT THE EQUIPMENT

When you tour a gym, make sure that the equipment is relatively new and clean. A good gym should have body balls, BOSU trainers, free weights, and a safe, non-slip floor to work out on. See that they have a variety of cable machines in place that has adjustable cables to maximize exercise combinations.

The best equipment I have ever used is called Human Sport, made by Star Trac (www.startrac.com). It's a series of six cable machines designed for a multitude of different exercises. For example, the Human Sport chest machine allows for a chest press movement as well as a pec fly movement. Both of these exercises can be performed in a seated or standing position, and single arm or both arms at once. The Human Sport leg machine allows for four separate movements that work all the muscles surrounding the leg. The exercises are done in a standing position with comfortable bars to hang onto for support and focus. Not only are the muscles in the front of the leg isolated, the groin muscles (inside the thigh), the gluteus (outside of the bum) and the hamstrings (back of the leg) are targeted as well. Over the six years of using the Human Sport with clients, I was constantly amazed at the brilliance and forethought that went into the design of these machines. If you find a fitness center that has similar equipment, you will know that it is the type of gym you are looking for. Also, the personal trainers there will undoubtedly be well versed in up-to-date weight resistant techniques and have a good understanding of corrective exercises.

CHECK OUT THE LOCKER ROOMS

Check out the locker rooms. If the rooms aren't extremely spacious and don't have waterfall shower heads in the showers, it's not the end of the world. What you really want to focus on is that they are clean.

At my gym on Salt Spring Island, we did not have room for co-ed change rooms and showers. Instead, we offered co-ed bathrooms and two separate shower rooms, and the majority of space was taken up by equipment and space for free weight exercises. At first, it seemed that this might be a barrier for customers who wanted co-ed change rooms. However, once people used our equipment and spent an hour with a personal trainer, they quickly changed their minds about their original priorities. Even still, when you try out a gym, take a change of clothes and use the change room and shower before making a final decision. This can give you a better feel of the facility accommodations for showering at the gym. Getting a preview of the full experience you will have every time you use the gym is essential in helping you to make a final decision.

CHECK OUT THE PERSONAL TRAINERS

Next, notice whether or not the personal trainers are doing creative exercises and stretches with their clients, which can be a reflection of how enthusiastic and interested the trainers are to work at the facility. Is there space for floor exercises? Are body balls being used routinely instead of benches? Take your time making a decision about joining a gym. Don't get caught up in the flashy, compelling sales pitch, no matter how cute the sales rep is. Gyms with great equipment and enthusiastic trainers working with a wide variety of age groups are the priority.

Approach with caution any facility or program that makes weight loss the selling feature. Maintaining an ideal body mass index is very important to your overall health, but it is essential to reduce or prevent pain syndromes and strengthen weak muscles before beginning a vigorous exercise program. While this initial training period will result in a healthier body composition, it should not, at first, be the main goal. Permanent weight loss will only occur through exercise and calorie reduction, and exercise can only occur if the body is healthy and free from injury. If you are deconditioned or new to exercise, it is essential to start slowly and listen to your body. Booking sessions with a personal trainer, and only working out within that session for the first few weeks or months will help prevent injuries and establish good exercise habits.

Joining the Gym/Signing Up

The International Health and Racquet Sports Association (IHRSA) is an international organization that has a code of conduct for its members. If you notice that the club you are joining is a member of the association, count it a very positive indication of the club's integrity toward members. The IHRSA has a great website with information about the association and an outline of the code of conduct:

+ Treat each member as if the success of the club depends on that individual alone.
+ Systematically upgrade professional knowledge and awareness of new developments in the industry.

+ Design facilities and programs with members' safety in mind.

+ Continue to increase the value and benefits of services and programs.

+ Provide public service programs to expand awareness of the benefits of regular exercise and sport.

+ Refrain from illegal activities and deceptive sales practices.

+ Deliver what is promised.

+ Conduct the business in a manner that commands the respect of the public for our industry and the goals for which we strive.

The code of conduct also states that it is important not to purchase a lifetime membership at any fitness club as memberships should never be for more than three years as the longevity of the club is undetermined and, as a result, selling lifetime memberships can be considered an illegal practice.

When you are asked to sign a contract, it is important to look at the fine print and find a clause that allows you to cancel your membership. The best rate is usually based on signing up for twelve months, which means that the club is giving you an advance for the annual membership and in return you agree to make monthly payments. If you decide to stop using the gym at some point during the year, you are still expected to continue paying the monthly fee until the end of the contract. Most contracts have a penalty clause for early cancellation, so before agreeing to have money taken directly from your bank account or credit card, you need to be clear on the rules for early cancellation.

Purchasing a gym membership is both a monetary commitment and a time commitment. Unless you use the gym regularly over an extended period of time, you will not see the expected results. *Using* the gym is the only way to get your money's worth. If you find that you are not using your membership, find a way to get back into the gym. Book a session with a trainer, read an inspirational book, find a friend to go with, or put the workout into your schedule at work or at home and stick to it. Remember to put yourself first. You are worth it.

The other way to purchase a membership is to pay up front for the entire year, which means that you don't have to worry about making monthly payments. Sometimes gyms offer short-term three-month or six-month contracts. Often, gyms will offer different types of memberships based on the needs of the population, including special rates for couples or families. If you take extended trips throughout the year, investigate the type of membership that would suit your schedule.

When you sign up, you will need to fill out a health questionnaire and discuss it with a qualified individual who can determine your readiness for exercise. If an individual has two or more risk factors for metabolic disorder, many gyms may ask for a doctor's note indicating that you are ready for an exercise program, along with any contraindications or concerns the physician may have. Risk factors include age, high blood pressure, high cholesterol, being overweight or having excess body fat (measured with a body composition analyzer and/or calipers), smoking, and a family history of heart disease. For example, a male over 45 is considered at a higher risk for heart disease, especially with a family history, while a female with a family history is not considered to be at a higher risk until she is over 55. The reason for this difference is that estrogen provides protection against heart disease, an effect that is not relevant to men. Once women go through menopause, they lose the protective effect of estrogen and their risk increases.

Remember that more women die of heart disease than from cancer, strokes, or COPD (chronic obstructive pulmonary disease), and heart disease is the number one killer of both men and women in North America. Women rarely survive a heart attack, whereas men are more likely to survive their first incident.

Owners and operators of fitness facilities are running a business in a time when people are still active later in life and therefore they need to create awareness of the risk of heart failure during intense exercise. The heart is a muscle that needs exercise in order to function properly, just like any other muscle in the body, but it is important to start slowly with a moderate aerobic exercise program to improve the condition of the heart muscle.

The muscles that make up our lungs need the same consideration. Being de-conditioned means that your heart and lung muscles will not work efficiently, which can make you feel weak and vulnerable if you start a vigorous exercise program before your body is conditioned.

Be aware that the first few weeks of exercising can make you feel worse before you feel better, but do not give up! Many things can go wrong at the beginning of a lifestyle change. You might get the flu, someone in the family might have a crisis, the family pet could get sick and require many trips to the vet, all of which could consume time and energy you had been hoping to put into exercising.

Even if there are no unforeseen circumstances that prevent you from going to the gym, it is easy to get distracted, feel too tired, and lose momentum during the first month of your membership. It seems to take about six months to develop a healthy habit and about six days to develop an unhealthy habit.

Beginning a regular exercise routine takes a sizeable investment of time and energy. Most people are unaware of all the difficulties that they will encounter at this stage of becoming a habitual exerciser. Be prepared. At my gym, we informed everyone that the first rule of exercise is that you do not have to love it or like it. Exercise is all about gaining and maintaining a level of fitness that allows you to do the things that you love. If exercise happens to be your passion, wonderful, but for 90 percent of the population it is not. The statistics are pretty clear: only 20 percent of the population will join a gym, less than 30 percent of the population will break a sweat from exercise during the year, and more than 60 percent of the adult population is overweight. I recently read an article that discussed surgery as a means of dealing with the morbidly obese, which are individuals who weigh at least two to three times a normal weight for their height and bone structure. The article stated that there are over a million morbidly obese adults in Canada. That is more than the total population of the province of Saskatchewan. I take this to mean that, generally, people do not like to exercise. This barrier to exercise needs attention, now and in the future, by everyone involved in the health and wellness field, as well as those who can make public policies that help diminish the barriers. If you don't love exercise, you're in good company, but you can't let that stop you from giving your body what it needs to be healthy.

Healthy Habits and Routine

Keep in mind that if you are new to exercise or it has been a while since you have had regular exercise (six months or more), then even one hour a week is a 100 percent increase in exercise time. Going three times in the first week translates into a 300 hundred percent increase. As I stated in a previous chapter, less is more when beginning any new exercise routine. If you can make it to the gym consistently once a week for a month, you will find it easier to bump it up to twice a week in the second month. Once you are easily able to get to the gym twice a week for a month, going three times a week will be the next step.

Our bodies function in a completely different manner than our brains. If you miss a week to go on vacation, the body does not go on vacation. The body will respond by putting an end to all the positive physiological changes that were a result of exercise. If you take a lengthy break from exercising (either for a holiday or due to unforeseen circumstances), when you eventually get back to a routine you will be starting all over again. This is a biological fact and can lead to a lot of frustration and misunderstanding. I have experienced people complaining that they could not see results and, therefore, gave up their gym membership when they actually did not even use the gym or did so very rarely.

We are so accustomed to making excuses, excuses that we start to actually to believe, but the body hears no excuses. Keep going, even if you are forced to take a break from the gym. If you can't get to the gym for some reason, walk, try a different exercise program, resist sitting for long periods, and be aware that you may experience sore muscles when you start up again. Don't despair over the muscle soreness as it is over quickly and is a sign that your muscles are reacting by getting stronger. Sore muscles are a good thing as it means a stronger more resilient body.

You can eliminate much of the stress of engaging in an exercise routine by doing some simple math. This is a great calculation: currently, you are not doing any exercise, which is equal to zero hours a year. You start doing an hour a week, which is 52 hours a year. After a while, you decide to exercise twice a week, which is 104 hours a year. By now, you are feeling fabulous so you bump it up to three times a week, which is 156 hours a year. Congratulations! You have gone from zero to 156 hours a year with very little change to your lifestyle. As an added bonus, if you consume the same amount of calories that you always have, you will lose a few pounds of body fat. In a year, your clothes will be looser rather than tighter, the latter being the unfortunate experience for the majority of the population. Consider that after ten years of three times a week you have accumulated 1560 hours of exercise time! Now you can enjoy all the benefits of dedicating over 1500 hours to exercise in your schedule. You feel better, look better, and you are in a better mood.

You sleep better and handle stress better. You're not having so much anxiety and your body works better physically and mentally. Now look at the total cost: gym memberships can be as low as $300 a year; after ten years you have invested somewhere between three and five thousand dollars, which is equivalent to the cost of a new set of furniture or a two-week Mediterranean cruise. The investment is a minuscule amount when compared to the benefits.

OVERCOMING INJURY/ PERSONAL TRAINING

If you have a specific foot or lower body orthopedic concerns, a consultation with a healthcare professional about footwear and proper exercises is a necessity. Everybody is unique and has a different health history. If you have any concerns, please have a discussion with your family doctor or another specialist before starting your exercise program.

Keep in mind that exercise is not always a magic bullet. There is no guarantee that exercise will solve all the problems involved with a medical condition. I can assure you, however, that lack of exercise will not help you get better, and in the long term, not exercising may cause your condition to worsen. As long as you have a well-designed exercise program and access to good equipment, you will realize the many positive benefits of regular exercise.

Be patient and seek the advice of a positive and proactive healthcare provider who encourages exercise and physical activity. Once cleared by your physician to start exercising after recovering from an illness or injury, seek out a personal trainer who has experience working with clients with specific needs. Make sure you have made a good connection with the trainer before you work with them long-term. As I previously stated, a professional will never be upset if they are not the right choice for a client at any given time in their exercise life. I had many clients switch to other trainers in my gym. At first, it was a little bit of a blow to the old ego, but I was quick to realize that having a choice is better for the clients and better for the trainers. Personal training is all about the human connection, and it is essential to begin an exercise program feeling comfortable and relaxed.

Pack a Gym Bag

Once you have located a few fitness facilities that are potentially a good fit, put some workout clothes and new running shoes in a bag and head to the gym for a free introductory workout. Make sure you have a separate bag for your gym gear. Keep it filled with all the essentials for your workout, and place it where it is visible by the front door. There are many companies that sell gym bags, which can be found in all shapes and sizes, and although they are a little more expensive, Lululemon (www.lululemon.com) is a great resource for such accessories. They have even designed a bag to separate your sweaty clothes from the rest of your gear at the end of your workout. Trust me, this is a great feature.

Once you start going to the gym, you will inevitably end up with sweaty clothes and extra laundry, so it is a good idea to have more than one outfit in case you are unable to wash your clothes right away. Remove all barriers to exercise right from the start. Forgetting your gym bag, not washing your gym clothes, or not having the right gear should not be an excuse. After all, you would not go camping without a tent, sleeping bag, cooking utensils, and matches to light a fire or cook stove. There is a reason for the enduring boy scout's motto: be prepared.

FOOTWEAR IS THE BASE OF THE GYM BAG

While you are out looking at gym bags, stop by an athletic shoe store and try on some new running shoes. The whole conversation about running shoes is lengthy and involved. Change has been constant over the last twenty years in the fitness industry, and evidence of these changes can be found most clearly in the evolution of running shoes. When Nike designed and sold their first running shoe many years ago, it was a revolution. I still remember purchasing my first fully-cushioned, white mesh Nike runners when I was in twelfth grade. They were beautiful and comfortable, albeit bulky.

Now, when I look down at my soft, brightly colored, thin-soled running shoes, it is hard to believe that, at one time, joggers wore shoes with soles over an inch thick that were built up with air and any other material to reduce impact. Then add the stark white color, and we looked like we were running on little clouds.

Eventually, the rate of running related injuries began to make a few savvy individuals question the wisdom of all that shoe cushioning. This investigation is the premise for *Born to Run* (Christopher McDougall, 2009), a great interesting and inspiration book about the history of the running shoe and how the concept of barefoot running became recognized as superior to the white clouds we had been trained to buy.

McDougall describes in detail the different features of the running shoe, the history of the running shoe, proper training programs for runners, and how their choice of running shoe effects joggers and runners, especially during long-distance events. Basically, McDougall points out that our feet were meant to be used. Our feet were designed to be used for running and to feel the ground when we run, so when we pad our feet with material to protect our joints from the impact of running, it actually has the opposite effect of what we once thought to be true. Barefoot running or wearing minimalist shoes protects our bodies from injury because our feet can work properly, the way they are meant to work. Without heavily padded shoes, we can maintain proper biomechanics, which keeps our joints in proper alignment. Yes, there is a case founded on science that thick running shoes can cause poor biomechanics while running, jogging, or even walking.

Coincidentally, even before I had read the book, I was encouraging my clients and members to work out in stocking feet. Some of my clients would show up to work out with shoes that were more like an ankle cast. After inserting their orthotics into their hard army-like shoes, they could barely walk, let alone attempt some balancing exercises. To make their workout comfortable and productive, I suggested they leave their shoes under the bench and work out shoe-free, just for an hour. For some, this was like asking them to cut off an arm. "But I was told to never, ever walk around in bare feet; even my slippers have orthotics," was the type of incredulous response I had to get used to. After some cajoling that was like convincing a cat to climb out of a tree, I usually got my way, and the results were amazing. Clients noticed reduced knee pain, improved balance, and less joint pain overall.

Most gyms have a clean shoe only policy and no bare feet allowed, which is practical and reasonable for everyone's safety and personal hygiene issues. Fortunately, most athletic shoe stores stock running shoes that mimic being barefoot while providing the hygiene and basic protection of shoes.

You may have noticed these strange shoes that look like gorilla feet showing up in public places. These shoes caught my eye and prompted me to investigate, leading me to realize that there is a lot more to the feet than most people understand. Humans have a large number of proprioceptors, which are cells that are part of the nervous system that sends information to the brain to indicate where the body is in space at any given time. These are located on the bottom of our feet, not, as I have regularly told my clients, on the bottom of our asses where when we are sitting there is not much information going to the brain and this can lead to many pain-causing postural deviations.

Basically, when we sit, the proprioceptors on the bottom of our feet are on an extended coffee break, and after their break, they are very slow to get back to work. Proprioceptors are little microsensors that are located in our extremities that send signals to our brain. These signals help the brain figure out where the body is in space and this is very important in balance and agility. The more you challenge your balance, the faster these sensors send information to your brain to correct where the body is in space. This quick correction can prevent accidents.

Proprioceptors have evolved to function while the body is upright, not sitting or lying down. This is just one more reason to stay upright. Not only are we a sitting culture, we also have designed our physical world to make moving more efficient, resulting in less work for the body. Elevators, escalators, cars, and comfortable furniture, to name a few, are modern conveniences that have led to less work for the foot muscles and which can have a potentially negative effect on the entire body.

One of the reasons that minimalist shoes are beneficial is that when you are upright, these shoes force the muscles of the feet to work harder, and at the same time, the proprioceptors on the bottom of the feet are far more sensitive to changes in foot pressure leading to better posture and a quicker reaction time in unstable environments.

Muscles in the feet need to be the strongest muscles in our body to withstand the load of our bodyweight, which is placed on the relatively small surface area of the soles. If the feet become weak, we are prone to tripping, falling and injuries of the ankles and knees. It is essential to create situations and partake in activities that challenge these muscles. One way to go about this is to design environments such as standing computer desks, incentives to park farther away from the office, limited access to elevators, fitness facilities within office buildings, paths that are designed for walking meetings that force us onto our feet, and keeping those muscles working as often as possible. This is where the benefits of the barefoot running shoe or minimalist shoe comes in. Compared to wearing supportive shoes, especially hard-topped shoes with orthotics, these shoes make sure that when you're on your feet, the muscles are working as hard as possible. Minimalist shoes are available in an array of colors and styles. The ten-toe gorilla look is not necessary. Nike now makes a shoe called Nike Free, which is essentially a barefoot running shoe that comes in varying degrees of support. It is important to break into these shoes gradually if you are running or walking in them, but for a one-hour, weight-resistant workout, they are ideal. My staff was persuasive in selling the barefoot idea to our clients, and soon we had a gym full of members wearing brightly colored minimalist shoes. We told our clients that they would feel better and joked that they would look ten years younger. We inspired them to buy new, hip running shoes to help them to get moving and to feel young and vigorous, and to become mentors for their friends and families.

There are a lot of opinions about athletic shoes and orthotics. If you are new to exercising, have lower body joint issues, or are planning to participate in a variety of activities such as running, dancing, cycling, walking, weight training, or aerobics, you may need different shoes for each activity. Be sure to ask your family doctor for advice on the best footwear if you have injuries or chronic pain syndrome. It is never wrong to ask the advice of different experts on shoes and orthotics before making the final purchase. Remember, fit, comfort, price, color, and the appropriate shoe for the chosen activity need to be on the checklist and crossed off when you shop for active-wear shoes.

So, plan to spend an afternoon shopping and getting that gym bag ready. Remember the Boy Scout motto, *be prepared?* Time spent preparing is well worth it and will be indispensable in easing you into your new healthy lifestyle.

WORKOUT CLOTHES

Once you have a gym bag and a pair of running shoes, it is time to purchase the gym outfit. There are many sports stores to choose from, but my personal favorites are Lululemon and Sport Chek. The style of exercise clothing has changed dramatically over the last twenty years as exercise has become mainstream. People wear gym clothes in public, before and after hitting the gym, so that has affected the style of workout attire.

The type of fabric used in activewear has improved as well. Lycra, for example, is lighter, breathes better, and is generally much more comfortable than cotton. Due to the improvements in and rise in popularity of workout clothing, Vancouver, the birthplace of Lululemon, is now rated as one of the worst dressed cities in North America! At the same time, Vancouver is one of the fittest cities in North America, which suggests that many Vancouverites favor fitness-chic over fashion. I am thrilled that people are recognizing the value of exercise and investing in the right clothes to make the experience that much more enjoyable, even if it means being labeled worst-dressed.

One of my pet peeves left over from owning a gym, is the big, thick, cotton t-shirt that people show up in that have things written on the back of it such as *volunteer* or *something-something conference* 1991. One of my first goals with a new client who walks in like this is to have them wear a tighter, lighter-weight t-shirt, preferably a black tank top or something equally simple and sleek. Not only does the client feel more comfortable, but the trainer can see how they are moving to correct their form, creating a much more effective workout.

I have witnessed the beginning of the transformation of many of my clients with the acquisition of new, attractive work-out clothes. Then, when they picked up dumbbells and ran on the treadmill, they completed the transformation. They felt and looked fabulous and the right attire brought it all together. It's like beautiful dishes and cutlery set on the table to make the dinner taste that much better.

One day I had to tell one of my clients that his oversized t-shirt and baggy shorts, that he had clearly pulled out of the dark forgotten recesses of his closet, weren't doing anything for his self-esteem. The following week he showed up in new shorts, shirt, and shoes. They fit well and were color coordinated. That same client lost 30 pounds training at the gym, and even now, when I see him, he is still wearing great workout clothes. What you choose to wear and present yourself in can have an enormous effect on how you feel and what you achieve. A word of caution: if you are currently overweight, hold off on too many purchases as your size and shape will change after six months of exercise. What a treat to have to buy smaller sized clothes in a few months' time! That is one of the many rewards of engaging in a healthier lifestyle.

LADIES, TAKE CARE OF YOUR GIRLS

Another important and somewhat complex issue is finding suitable bra tops. If you have not yet purchased a sports bra, this is the time to do some research and choose a brand and fit that works for you., Make sure you have several in rotation.

For women, the sports bra is an essential part of the exercise outfit. Having attended seminars on sports bras given by athletic companies, I have been amazed at all the issues surrounding support and comfort. Fortunately, there are many fabrics, designs, and colors to choose from. According to Warner's Bras, a large manufacturer of women's bras, the average chest size has gone from a B cup to a C cup, which is a result of the weight gain we see in the general population, making it more important than ever to have good, supportive sports bra. Besides making exercise more comfortable, a well-chosen sports bra can make you look slimmer and feel less self-conscious in the gym or exercise class.

By now, you should feel educated and inspired to pick out a new workout outfit, a new pair of workout shoes, and the right kind of sports bag to pack it all. The next step is to hit the gym!

Making the Commitment and Getting through the First Week

A major issue surrounding exercise is the amount of time that is needed to get healthy and improve your fitness level. There are minimum exercise requirements to be healthy and to reduce the risk of degenerative diseases, but to be fit or to improve fitness levels the whole commitment changes. For maximizing health benefits, I recommend working out for one hour, twice a week, using weight resistant exercises and completing four hours of cardio at moderate intensity per week.

If you want to improve your fitness level or compete in an athletic event, more time is required and intensity will increase, but the critical factor is to remember that *less is more in the beginning of any positive lifestyle change*. If you are new to exercise and can get to the gym twice a week for a year with only a few breaks, you will easily become committed to your workout sessions.

If a non-exerciser starts out by going to the gym three to five times a week, they will usually be gone after a month as they become overwhelmed with the whole process. Then, when they fail to get to the gym often enough, they suffer post-exercise muscle pain or do not see instant results, and they give up. After training hundreds of clients and observing thousands of people and their exercise habits, it is easy to see patterns of behavior. According to the 2009 Heart Disease and Statistics report, 62 percent of Americans over the age of eighteen lead completely sedentary lifestyles. This is an amazing stat, given the amount of education and information that we have on the benefits of regular exercise. Just think, if you can manage to work out a minimum of two days a week for 60-minutes a session, you will increase your fitness and be twice as active as 62 percent of the population.

Now that you have found the perfect gym and have signed up for more than a month, let's talk about some of the details that will help you maximize your gym time and get through those first few weeks.

A LOOK AT YOUR FIRST WEEK AT THE GYM

Showing up early for your first training and orientation session will give you time to change and be relaxed before you begin to use the exercise equipment. Make sure you strictly follow your trainer's advice in the first month, as that is the time when most people give up. You do not want to develop poor habits or form during your first sessions and your trainer will help keep you from doing that if you follow their instructions.

If you are uncomfortable around large crowds, book your sessions during a quiet time in the gym. This will minimize your anxiety and help you focus on your exercises and body, rather than looking around at all the people.

During the first week, only go to the gym a maximum of three times, allowing your body and brain to get used to the new routine without being overwhelmed. While you should be prepared for some muscle soreness after your first few sessions, it is important not to overdo it. Starting out slowly and continuing steadily is the most important part of exercising. Remember the point of the tortoise and the hare fable is that *slow and steady wins the race.*

When you experience delayed onset muscle soreness or DOMS as it is technically referred to, it will be two to three days after your workout. This is why it is best to have only a few exercise sessions during your first week. DOMS is the worst at the beginning of your exercise program. Don't be put off by the soreness in your muscles or think the muscles are injured. Expect some soreness and rest assured that it will not continue. DOMS takes a few days to go away, and although it is a bit uncomfortable, it is a normal physiological reaction when the muscles are deconditioned.

It is imperative that you avoid injury at this stage of your exercise program, which is another reason to have an expert to guide you. If you have an existing injury or a severe restriction because of a past injury to any joints or muscles or have restrictions because of surgery, it is extremely important to relay this information to your trainer. Having had a proper interview and assessment with your trainer, creativity, and sound exercise principals will guide you through a great exercise program that meets all your specific needs.

Remember that your compliance is essential. Be present and attentive while learning a new skill and continue to exercise with awareness to avoid injury and maximize your results. It will take at least six months to really notice an increase in strength. It will take the same amount of time to realize a reduction in pain if you have been injured in the past or have had surgery due to an injury or arthritis. This is where patience pays off. If at any time during your exercise program you experience sharp pain that does not go away or a definite reduction in muscular strength, you need to talk to your doctor, and the sooner the better, as quitting is not an option.

WORKING OUT IF YOU TRAVEL

If you travel frequently, it is essential to continue your exercise program while you are away. Investigate the gyms available in the hotel or near the hotel, and make sure your work days include time for a workout. Depending on where you travel, hotels often have an affiliation with a personal training business and allow you the option to prepay for sessions before you arrive, guaranteeing that you will fit your workouts into your schedule. Traveling, especially for work, can be very stressful on the body, but time away from your hectic home life can be an opportunity to focus on working out and maybe doing something different than you would at home. Plus, a personal trainer often knows about local recreation better than most tour guides. Even airports are starting to provide workout facilities for travelers: Goodlife Fitness has opened a gym at the Toronto airport, a sign of a future in which fitness will be readily available in places where people are forced to spend their time sitting and waiting. Wherever you are, getting that workout in is all a matter of planning and creativity.

If you're traveling for recreation or holiday, it is equally important to keep up a regular exercise routine. When you are booking your trip, consider destinations where you can continue to exercise. For example, cruise ships offer many exercise classes and weight lifting equipment, and often there are personal trainers on board. Most resort destinations offer similar services. Even if you're traveling somewhere that doesn't offer these facilities, it is possible to plan ahead for walks and hikes. Guide books for the area usually feature hiking trails and public parks for walking. Some cities have beautiful waterfronts that are a great place to walk or run.

Many of my clients planned active holidays in conjunction with activities such as walking or cycling tours. There are many beautiful destinations such as New Zealand that are famous for hiking or walking. My daughter recently traveled to Nepal and hiked to the base camp of Mt. Everest. One of the best experiences clients have reported was cycling through the south of France. No matter what your destination, do your best to make exercise a priority. If your trip does not allow for much exercise time, be sure to book a personal training session at your gym during the week that you arrive home. This is a good trick to be motivated to get back into a regular routine. Traveling can be a significant barrier to exercise, and it takes some people weeks or even months to get back to the gym after arriving home. Don't let that happen. Make sure exercise is on the list of priorities to attend to once you arrive back home.

Eating and Drinking

On top of all that, once you start working out, you're going to have to start paying more attention to getting the right nutrition and staying hydrated. Make sure that you include a bottle of water in your gym bag. Water consumption has become a hot topic over the last few years. Most people do not consume enough water during the day, instead choosing coffee, tea, or drinks with a high sugar content. We require at least eight, eight-ounce (240 ml) glasses of water a day to stay healthy. The brain requires the most water of any organ. With even slight dehydration, the brain can slow down enough to cause memory loss. Another issue is the fact that when we feel hunger it is often that we are dehydrated. It is very important to drink water throughout the day and avoid beverages that are high in sugar. The extra calories are unnecessary and simple sugars can interfere with insulin production, ultimately contributing to adult onset diabetes. The amount of pop and sweetened juice that North Americans consume is staggering. At one time, one of our local grocery stores on Salt Spring Island reported their biggest selling items, by volume, were pop and ice cream. The solution is to not buy it and don't drink it. When we are becoming dehydrated during the day and our brains are not fully functioning, it is often far easier to grab the wrong food and drink. Prevention is key here. Plan ahead for your water consumption and always drink more while you are exercising.

FUEL YOUR BODY AND REMEMBER YOU ARE WHAT YOU EAT

If you have poor eating habits, now is the time to make changes. Eating poor quality food has a negative effect on your overall health, but continuing to consume calorie-rich, nutrient-poor foods will almost certainly shorten your time at the gym.

Nutrition is one of the most poorly understood subjects amongst the general population. Many healthcare providers do not even understand the fundamentals of good nutrition. Then add in the billion-dollar supplement industry that produces a product for every problem known to mankind and, according to them, with the right supplement, you can instantly become smarter, stronger, better looking, and happier. Recently, scientific evidence has been released confirming that the consumption of too many supplements and in too great a quantity may cause more harm than good. With that in mind, it is always a good idea to consume high-quality, nutrient-dense foods to get your recommended daily allowance of micronutrients (vitamin and minerals) and macronutrients (proteins, carbohydrates, and fats).

MACRO-NUTRIENTS ARE THE MOST IMPORTANT
NUTRIENTS WHEN HITTING THE GYM

The body needs *carbohydrates*, *proteins*, and *fats* to exist, and it needs them in the right proportion to enable you to exercise properly without crashing. By crashing, I am referring to the state that many people experience due to insufficient calorie consumption before their workout. They start by shaking, then going pale, then asking to sit down, and ultimately leaving early to go home and lie down. When questioned, it becomes obvious that either they have not eaten enough food or they are on some weird diet that restricts calories or macro-nutrients. It only takes one or two crashes to get people to start preparing their bodies with the appropriate pre-workout meals. If you are well nourished, you can give 100 percent during your workout. With proper nutrition, you'll maximize your time at the gym, which translates into fewer trips for the same great results.

Carbs

Carbohydrates are the sugars in our diet. They are either simple sugars such as granulated sugars found in cakes and cookies or complex carbs found in low glycemic foods such as vegetables and oatmeal. It is a good idea to research the glycemic index of different foods and choose mainly low glycemic foods like fruit, vegetables, oatmeal, and beans. As a rule of thumb develop the habit of always choosing the apple over the chocolate bar. Your body stores carbohydrates in the muscles in order to provide fuel for the muscles during activity. Restricting your carbohydrate intake to a very small percentage of your diet means that exercise will quickly tire you out. You should be getting at least 50 percent of your total caloric intake from carbohydrates, preferably low glycemic foods with the occasional cheat (like a cookie or chocolate.) As you may know, our muscles burn calories simply to live. Having more muscle means burning more calories every day. Therefore, you will burn extra calories as you put on extra muscle. In essence, when you add muscle mass to your body, you are creating a bigger machine that needs more fuel. This means when you have more muscle, you can consume more calories without experiencing weight gain. In order to gain this muscle mass, you have to do progressive weight resistant exercising. Sitting and contemplating is not a substitute! It is a common recommendation to consume a small meal that is comprised of mostly low-glycemic foods about an hour before exercising There are many excellent cookbooks and nutrition books written by registered dietitians that provide ideas for a pre-workout meal.

If you find that working out is sometimes a last minute decision, be sure to carry fruit and healthy bars with you at all times. I always keep a Clif Builder's Bar and a banana in my gym bag - just in case.

Protein

The next macro-nutrient to look at is protein. There are as many beliefs around eating protein as there are non-dairy beverages at the local coffee shop. On Salt Spring Island, we have many vegetarians and vegans who won't consume animal products, not even honey. Organic raw food vegans really have a limited choice when it comes to dining out. In other words, removing animal protein from the diet can limit your choices for protein.

The decision to reduce or completely stop consumption of meat products is often made for reasons other than health. I find it commendable to be concerned about the future of the planet and to respect animal welfare. Unlike carbohydrates, you do not need to consume a large percentage of protein in your diet, but you do need the right amount of high-quality protein every day to keep your body running at its best. High-quality protein for meat eaters is from sources rich in protein that exclude saturated fats. It's healthier to choose salmon and skinned chicken breast over T-bone steaks and bacon. For vegetarians, healthy protein choices include beans and brown rice mixed with a healthy variety of vegetables over pasta and Alfredo or white sauce. Vegans choose only plant-based protein sources, consuming tofu and nuts, rather than eggs and dairy products.

It is generally accepted that your diet should be 15 to 25 percent protein. Imagine that protein is to your body what oil is to your car. If you have poor quality oil that is dirty or contaminated in your engine, there will be many problems with the way your car runs, and eventually, a breakdown will occur.

Proteins are made up of two kinds of amino acids: essential and non-essential. Essential amino acids cannot be produced by the human body, and since they are important for proper bodily functions, they must be consumed in our diet. If you need 100 grams of protein per day and you only consume 80 grams, your body will breakdown or tap into its own muscles as a source to harvest the amino acids needed for physiological functions that keep you alive.

There are many different opinions on how much protein each person needs per day. A good rule of thumb is one gram per kilogram of body weight per day for someone who is completely sedentary. This means that a 50 kg sedentary female needs to consume 50 g of high-quality protein per day. This formula varies depending on the age, health status, and activity level of the person. An active 50 kg woman may require 100 g of protein per day.

Protein requirements also change between the sexes, especially as men will put on more muscle than women of the same age and health status. It is a good idea to consult a dietician or nutritionist before starting an exercise program. There are potential problems with increasing animal proteins for many people, and it is important to have the right mix of foods if your diet is entirely vegetarian. Most people consult a financial expert about their money, so why not consult an expert about your nutritional requirements to keep that engine running as smoothly as possible.

Fats

Then we move onto the subject of fats, and it is a big subject – literally. Over 60 percent of North Americans are over-weight, a result of high-fat meals and a gradually increasing standard portion size. Calories from fat should make up 15 to 25 percent of our diet. While the Atkins Diet touts an intake of 30 percent fat, which is too high to be healthy, going too far the other way is not good either. Consuming only 10 to 25 percent fat, 25 percent protein, and 65 percent carbs is not only difficult, but you lose the benefits of good quality fats. The good quality fats that you should consume are in healthy food sources such as avocados, certain nuts, olives, certain oils, fish (particularly cold-water), flax seeds, flax oil, hemp seeds and hemp oils. As a generalization, in North America, we consume too much fat from the wrong sources, including high-fat meat products, which should be avoided at all costs. To your heart, the fat in that T-bone steak or hamburger and fries is like a small earthquake that is a warning of a bigger shock to come if that tectonic plate keeps moving or in the case of your heart, clogged arteries if saturated fat is continuously consumed. Instead, opt for a salad or mixed vegetables and a piece of fish. All processed foods should be avoided, particularly when there are plenty of tasty nutritional alternatives available.

Over the last fifteen years, there has been an increased emphasis on overweight and obese individuals but only relatively little conversation about the food industry's role in creating a desire for high-fat, low-nutrient foods. Despite movies such as *Super-Size Me* (2004) and *Food, Inc.* (2008), or books such as Michael Pollan's *The Omnivore's Dilemma* (2006) and Jonathan Safran Foer's *Eating Animals* (2009) that shed light on some of the large corporate food companies, the mainstream discussion centers around motivating overweight individuals to exercise and eat healthier foods. There is more discussion about giant oil companies and other corporations that have a negative effect on the environment than about the equally harmful corporate food culture.

It is time to become educated about our food, where it comes from, and who benefits from our purchases of food. Is it the farmers, the restaurants, the local grocery stores, or a large corporate food company that we support when we shop for groceries? Furthermore, it is time to become knowledgeable about the nutritional quality of the foods we choose to consume. In doing so, we are taking responsibility to maintain our health and pass knowledge of health on to the next generation.

Now, let's get back to the conversation about fats. When making choices about fat sources, consider that the type of fat that you ingest stays in the same form in the blood stream. For example, if you consume fats that are hard at room temperature, which are saturated fats like butter and lard, they remain saturated fats in your blood stream and can become part of the plaque that causes strokes and heart attacks. This is a key concept to keep in mind because fats are used for many important biological functions, most importantly as the building blocks of our cell membranes. Cell membranes have intricate biological functions, allowing substrates or nutrients to flow through the membrane into the cell, and waste products to flow out. The cell membrane is made up of the fats that we consume. If we eat mostly saturated fats, especially ones that are hard at room temperature, then those cell membranes will be stiff and less functional than cell membranes that are built from healthy fats like olive oil, nut oils such as walnut or sesame, and fats from plant sources like avocados, to name a few. The stiff cell will have difficulty performing its most basic task, which is allowing the flow of nutrients into the cell and waste products out of the cell. Imagine the pipes in your house. What if water could not flow in and sewage could not flow out? Healthy fats also have a positive effect on brain function, nerve function, hair, and skin. It is beneficial to get advice from a professional on how to incorporate the right amount of good quality fats into your diet on a daily basis.

You will benefit from this advice in many ways, even if you are sedentary. Of course, this book is written to inspire sedentary people to start exercising, but the main point is that everybody benefits from better eating habits.

5:

Building the Ultimate Muscle Machine: Weight Training

When we use the word *exercise*, we mean, simply, that our muscles are going to either move for a period of time or move a weight (body weight or external weight), or both. Muscles can be exercised through increased endurance (movement) or increased strength (moving weight). Other tissues in our bodies will benefit indirectly as a result of exercise, but the primary adaptations or changes take place in our muscles. The purpose of this chapter is to explain what muscle is and why we want to build and maintain this machine.

What Exactly is Muscle?

Muscle is a tissue that is attached to our bones by tendons and, as a result of this design, they move our skeleton. Ligaments attach bones to other bones and are not attached to muscles. This is an important distinction in terms of understanding injuries and the rationale behind a rehabilitation program.

Without muscle, our bones could not move and we would literally be nothing more than skin and bones!

Each one of our muscles causes an isolated movement at the bone or bones it is attached to. When a single body part moves, it is called an isolation exercise. Many muscles working together create whole-body movement, referred to as compound exercise. This is the fundamental difference, for example, between a pushup and a bicep curl. While a pushup causes most of the muscles in the body to engage, a bicep curl primarily targets the bicep (or upper-arm) muscle. In the pushup, you move at your ankle joint, knee joint, hip joint, back, shoulder joint, and elbow joint, compared to a simple bicep curl where the only movement is at your elbow joint.

It's no wonder that there continues to be confusion and speculation about what weight lifting routine is the best and why. It was not until relatively recently that weight resistant exercises were considered imperative to one's overall health. The first public health club opened in Santa Monica, California, in 1947. This was seven years before we even knew the scientific basis of the movement of muscle cells. Much of our understanding of weightlifting comes from new science and it takes time for scientific knowledge to filter down into mainstream understanding. Much of the weight lifting you see at your gym or in magazines comes from a more traditional understanding, which is a tradition that began long before science discovered, in 1954, how muscle fibers work to produce movement.

Basically, our physical form exists because of the way our muscles create action and the way they are attached to our bones. Muscles provide the foundation for our human form. They are the machine. Imagine the removal of muscles from the human body to be the equivalent of taking all the supportive metal frame out of a car. The end result would be something that could not function as a drivable car. Our muscles are beautiful, giving us our form and the ability to function. Celebrate your muscles, grow your muscles, look after your muscles. They are as precious as the air we breathe.

Muscles move because your brain sends an electric impulse to a muscle, or group of muscles, that causes a series of events. The end result is movement. Much of the motion of the human body is unconscious. About 90 percent of the time your body is moving without actually having to think about it. We would never get through the day if we had to think about every single movement we make. The fact that we move mostly without thinking about it is an example of evolution at its finest. Moving without having to think about it leaves our brains the freedom to focus on other activities.

General moving about is a totally different experience from weight lifting, which involves focus and concentration, both of which benefit your muscles and your brain. For some, lifting weights may be the first time they have ever focused on their muscles, concentrating on feeling their muscles working while they focus on movement. This can be exhausting for the new exerciser and for their nervous system.

Weight training will not only positively affect your muscles, but it will improve your nervous system, including the brain. Over time, everyday movements and activities of daily living (ADL) will be easier for your brain to perform unconsciously, thus freeing up precious energy for other pursuits. This is one of the fundamental principles behind exercise practices like yoga, Pilates, and dance. Proponents of these systems know that learning and practicing difficult movements changes the brain and reduces mental stress and anxiety. Science has caught up and has proven what the masters of the above activities already knew: use it or lose it. Remember that moving the body creates a more functional mind.

The body is a master at saving energy. When you stop moving, the body stops putting any energy into building muscle or conserving the existing muscle. This occurs very quickly. For an example, when you break a bone and have that limb immobilized, the muscles attached to that bone will start to get smaller and weaker within hours.

The body will not waste any energy on unused processes. However, the opposite is also true. If your body is being called to action, it immediately puts energy into making the muscles strong enough to meet those demands. If the demands are too extreme, injuries or general fatigue can occur. That is why a weight resistance program needs to be modest in the early stages to avoid injury and excessive fatigue.

To continue to increase strength, at some point, you must increase the amount of weight being lifted. If you are satisfied with your strength level, you may, instead, want to just focus on maintaining what you have. The nervous system will get used to a repetitive routine, so if you continue to do the same workout for more than a month, you may maintain strength levels, but continued progress will halt. For further results and to beat boredom, change your routine often. This can be accomplished by changing personal trainers, changing the order of the exercises, doing more or fewer sets, increasing the weights, and using completely different equipment The variables are endless. Remember that both the brain and the muscles must be constantly stimulated in different ways to keep your body in top condition. Changing your routine will promote the motivation and inspiration that will get you to the gym or to your next workout.

Aerobics versus Weight Training

Understanding the difference between weight training and cardio conditioning is essential as each one achieves very different outcomes. The goal of weight training is to increase the strength and power of muscles while cardio conditioning makes your muscles more efficient when using energy over long periods of time. Why do we need strength and power? Strength and power are both needed for many reasons. Being strong means less risk of injury. Any gain in muscle mass increases your metabolism, which results in burning more calories every day, even while you sleep. Bigger, stronger muscles equal more youthful hormones, which is the purest anti-aging system around. The stronger you are, the better you feel in your own skin, and this is reflected in your attitude toward life.

Another positive side effect of getting stronger muscles is stronger bones. Weight training significantly reduces the risk of osteoporosis. When you lift weights, your body receives a message that the weight is too much for your current bone strength, and in response, your brain sends out a signal to your bones to start the process of bone building. The opposite is true if you do not challenge your body with exercise. The body decides to stop wasting energy in the bone building department when the bones appear to be on holiday.

The Consequences of Being Sedentary

A sedentary body does not need much muscle, so what happens to the unused muscle? Muscle fibers are shut down, and at some point, these fibers disappear forever. Like factories that are no longer needed, they sit vacant until they are eventually bulldozed down. *Use it or lose it.* Lost muscle fibers are like downsizing to a condo once the kids leave. It's more efficient in terms of energy and expense, but when all the kids come home with grandchildren, there is less room and you can't create extra space. Trying to get active again after a time spent being sedentary is like the grandchildren coming home.

The permanent irreversible loss of muscle is a recognized medical condition called Sarcopenia. The reality is that everyone will lose up to 50 percent of their muscle between the ages of 20 and 90. However, lifting weights throughout your life can slow down the loss of muscle. For example, if you start off in your twenties with a good base of muscle (another reason to keep teenagers fit and healthy), and work out throughout your life, you may lose only 25 percent of your muscle. Working out is a huge insurance policy against age-related diseases. As a result of menopause, women are even more prone to muscle loss due to a decline in estrogen levels. Since muscle is metabolically active, women losing muscle during menopause can sometimes experience sudden weight gain. That said, an increase in body fat cannot be blamed entirely on menopause. It is also the result of a sedentary lifestyle that snowballs when the muscle is declining more rapidly than ever before. The bottom line is that for men and women alike, acquiring and maintaining muscle means a healthier, leaner, more vigorous body.

Many women shy away from lifting weights because they don't want big muscles. They see pictures of female body builders and are afraid of muscles popping and veins bulging out on their body. Some women prefer to emulate those super-skinny models with so little muscle that their bones protrude, supposedly representing beauty. The good news is that you do not have to get bigger just because you are stronger. Everyone will gain some mass as a result of lifting weights. This is a cause for celebration. The greatest fear of the general public should be their increased size from getting fatter, not from gaining muscle.

Many men are concerned about bulking up as well. Either they do not like the look or are competing in sports where strength to weight ratio is very important. If you follow a speed and power program, you will get stronger without bulking up. As an example, lifting heavy weights that you can only lift with correct form for less than five repetitions or lifting a given weight faster and becoming fatigued within 30 seconds, or performing body weight and balancing exercises to fatigue, slowly or quickly, or engaging in speed and agility training, like the 300-meter shuttle run (memories of high school PE) all help you gain strength without bulking up.

THE REASON YOU CAN WEIGHT TRAIN
WITHOUT BULKING UP

An untrained muscle, a muscle that has not been strengthened either through everyday activities or an exercise program, can only activate about 30 percent of its muscle fibers when needed, primarily because the nervous system has not been challenged and is not responsive to the demands placed on it. Conversely, a muscle that has been consistently exercised through everyday activities or an exercise program creates a nervous system that is in shape and responsive (in comparison to an untrained muscle). Therefore, up to 80 percent of the trained muscle fibers can be activated by the brain when needed. In other words, if you activate more muscle fibers in a given muscle, you don't need to get bigger muscles to do the job that is being demanded. The translation of that statement is that *big muscles are not necessarily stronger muscles, but trained muscles are definitely stronger muscles.*

The best example to illustrate this point is that of the superhuman strength some people have experienced in traumatic times such as when a small woman lifts a car in order to save someone's life. And there are many other extraordinary stories of human strength. What the journalists who report these stories don't include is the fact that those humans who do extraordinary feats tear muscles, tendons, and ligaments while performing those amazing feats. The super-human may even be hospitalized for extreme injuries after the feat. Under extreme stress, the body can activate muscle fibers that are untrained, but there is a cost. It takes time for a body to build strength and resiliency in connective tissues such as tendons, ligaments, and muscles. It is time to get the nervous system practiced at responding quickly to the demands of the body. However, once you have trained the muscle fibers and nervous system, the muscle fibers stick around. They are on call and available when you need them.

Once you are stronger and activating more muscle fibers, you will develop more insulin receptor sites on your muscle cells, making it easier for your body to minimize fat storage and stay lean. Muscular strength also translates into better posture. When muscles are strong they hold your body in a better postural position, which is very important to prevent wear and tear of your joints. Good posture can be achieved through educating yourself on techniques and benefits and through appropriate exercise selection. Maintaining correct body alignment increases energy and reduces pain syndromes such as lower and upper back pain. Most shoulder and neck troubles are relieved by improved posture as well.

Reducing pain and increasing energy makes activities of daily living (ADL) easier, and participating in fun, inspiring activities is the goal of an engaged life rather than simply using all of your energy just to get out of bed, get dressed, and accomplish a few basic chores.

Sheena's Beginner Weight Resistance Program

Do the following ten exercises, twice a week for two sets of 15 repetitions with a 60-second break between each set. This is a great program for eight weeks and then it needs to be changed. The order of exercises is important.

Warm-up on your favorite cardio machine for 15 to 30 minutes.

1. **Basic bodyweight squat** (make sure you have your form checked)
2. **Hamstring curl** using a machine
3. **Seated row**
4. Basic **chest press** using a machine
5. **Shoulder press** seated on a bench (palms face your body - elbows in)
6. A simple **triceps exercise**
7. A simple **bicep exercise**
8. **A plank** for the abdominal muscles - either on the knees for beginners or toes if you are strong, and hold for ten seconds times five reps. (Make sure a gym attendant demonstrates this exercise)

NOTE: This workout should not last longer than an hour.

Muscle is Nature's Art

Muscle gives us our shape and form and it is the machine that burns fuel and keeps us lean. It is the material that holds our skeleton together and creates hormonal conditions that promote healthy aging. Strong, fit muscle is the foundation of a great body, and gaining muscle and strength should be an integral part of a well-designed exercise program. Proper equipment and expert advice are essential to get results from your effort, which is another reason that you've chosen to join a fitness center that is home to modern equipment and knowledgeable staff. As a fitness guru, I need to express the fact that I love muscles. I love their strength, the way they look, the way they make us look in our clothes, the way they fight gravity, and the beauty and grace they give to our movements., I love how they assist us in accomplishing important tasks throughout the day, like unscrewing the lid from the jar without asking for help. Muscles are the fountain of youth and the provider of energy and strength to move us forward in this journey we call life. Have fun gaining your muscle! Take photos of your muscles. Kiss your bicep in front of the mirror occasionally and express gratitude for all the joy those muscles are going to bring to you.

6:

Aerobics Provide the Fuel for the Muscle Machine

While I write this chapter, I find myself reflecting on how much my aerobic fitness has contributed positively to my life. There have been many moments throughout my life where decisions have been made based on my energy level. My children would often ask to play one more game of tag, stay for another slide at the pool, play another round of ping pong, or build one more sandcastle on the beach. Many times I would feel tired with a cloud of fatigue about to roll in, then suddenly, I would get a little burst of energy and think *why not*. And then the fun would continue until someone was crying or hungry.

Every time I engaged in an activity that elevated my heart and made me sweat for more than 30 minutes, the effects on my life were remarkable. Think of those times when your partner wants to be engaged in relationship-building and you say, "No too tired." There are times when a friend needs help moving, a family member needs support during an appointment, children need exercise when they are wound up and house-bound, or a significant other wants to go for an evening walk instead of sitting on the couch together watching TV. All these little moments added together result in a life well- lived or a life watching others live.

The Magic Bullet for a Good Life

These moments added up to positive decisions being made because my fitness level is high and my energy and enthusiasm is parallel to my aerobic fitness. The benefits are enormous. When you have energy and enthusiasm because you feel well, life can be lived fully. Relationships can be created and sustained and events experienced instead of just watching life on a reality TV show.

As far as I am concerned, there is a magic bullet for living life, and it's called *get off the couch and move until you sweat and breathe hard*. How can we expect to function to our highest capacity if walking from our car to our house makes us tired? Sitting all day and sitting all evening makes us good at sitting, but that leaves out an entire category of activities that involve a higher fitness level. As we become physically fit, our energy level increases and we are able to experience more and do more and still feel good.

Exhaustion is often a result of being weak and deconditioned and is the not the normal state of the human body. On a scale of one to ten with the aerobically fit being a ten, most people are at a three. Work on being a ten and experience what being a ten is all about. Keep up with your endurance training program and notice how your enjoyment of life improves. The following chapter will discuss aerobics and the physiology and significance of this type of exercise. The message of becoming fit and staying fit will be motivating and empowering and recognized as a necessary part of enjoying life.

Remember that endurance training simply means that muscles are trained to be able to continue to contract and relax over a period of time with less effort than untrained muscles. An example of the effect of endurance training can be found in the action of stair climbing. If you are sedentary and have to climb up four flights of stairs, your leg muscles will most likely burn before you get to the top of the stairs. You may have to stop half way up to catch your breath, and at the top, you may feel wobbly and need to sit for a few minutes to recover. In contrast, if you have been jogging three times a week for 30 minutes a session for three months, your leg muscles will be used to taking in oxygen quickly and converting stored glucose into adenosine triphosphate (ATP), which is energy. This allows your muscles to contract and relax efficiently, meaning you would not have to stop at the top of the stairs to recover. If climbing four sets of stairs feels like a marathon, you know that your muscles are not being exercised aerobically. This is a great time to start an endurance training program.

Exercise Physiology Information for the Beginner

When you first start an exercise program or are coming back to exercise after a long sabbatical, it is important to understand a few basic concepts in exercise physiology to demystify all the conflicting information going around about the subject. First of all, aerobics, cardio, and endurance training mean the same thing to your muscles: moving your body enough to get your heart rate up past resting rate to at least 50 percent of your maximal heart rate (MHR), and keeping your heart rate at that level for at least 30 minutes (or for less time if your heart rate is closer to 80 percent of its MHR).

MAXIMAL HEART RATE (MHR)

Maximal heart rate is the maximum number of beats per minute that your heart can achieve. The absolute MHR varies with your age, gender, and to some degree your genetics, and can be measured in a variety of ways. The old school thinking in the scientific community is to set the absolute MHR of any human at their peak (18 to 25 years of age) at 220 beats per minute, then subtract their age. For example, the MHR of a forty-year-old would have been 180. As we age this number does, in fact, go down, but not necessarily by as much as one's age. The absolute accurate measure of your MHR requires a treadmill test, in a hospital, under the supervision of a cardiovascular specialist. In the meantime, it is important to have a fitness expert determine your training zone based on your age and health status, using a more accurate measure than the above.

Your training zone is the heart rate in beats per minute that you need to sustain for a given period of time in order to create all the positive effects that you are attempting to gain through exercise. I will be going into detail about these positive effects in the rest of this chapter.

When you are getting your heart rate up into the training zone, you may be sweating and breathing hard, but at the cellular level, you are training your muscles cells to break down the glucose and fat stored in the muscle cells, liver, and fat cells. Converting the substrates of glucose or fat into adenosine triphosphate (ATP) creates the energy needed to move your muscle fibers. This takes place in the mitochondria. Heat and carbon dioxide are by-products of this process. The heat makes you work up a sweat and the carbon dioxide ultimately gets released out through your lungs as the air you exhale. The oxygen from each breath of air you inhale gets transported to your muscle fibers through your blood. The oxygen goes into your muscle cells and combines with ATP. Keep in mind that the original decision to move created the need to increase breathing to get enough oxygen into the muscle cells to make more energy to keep moving.

What I find most interesting about this process is that plants do the exact opposite. They take in carbon dioxide to make energy to grow and expel oxygen as a byproduct. This is how plants and animals coexist on our planet in perfect harmony.

FUEL FOR AEROBIC EXERCISE

Now, it will be easier to understand why you have to eat food to fuel your muscles. As I mentioned above, glucose (made from the carbohydrates that you consume) and fat are both stored within your muscle cells as well as your liver and fat cells. The fat cells are located in various areas around your body, and not necessarily in places that you choose. These two fuels are taken into your mitochondria to be used as a source of energy. Think of it as being like throwing a log on the fire to heat the house.

As you get fitter and your aerobic capacity increases, your body naturally stores more glucose within the muscle cells. However, the body has limitations on how much glucose can be stored, and therefore, must rely on fats as a fuel source. It is good news, indeed, that we can give away our extra fat stores as fuel. Now, a fat molecule delivers over twice the energy of a glucose molecule. For example, the glucose stored in muscles of a 145- pound adult at 18 percent body fat will only allow for about 100 minutes of marathon running whereas the fat stored in the same adult will allow for five days of marathon running.

For those of us constantly battling the bulge, the great news is that once you start *and continue* a regular endurance exercise program you are training your mitochondria to use fat as a fuel source instead of relying mainly on glucose. As a matter of fact, once you reach a higher level of aerobic fitness and are able to participate in lengthy endurance activities without getting fatigued, your mitochondria use fat as fuel all day long, even outside of exercise time.

These physiological adaptations that the body makes as an individual become fitter – climbing the stairs without getting tired, burning more fat as an energy source all day long – have fantastic side effects. You will have more energy to do more of the things you love, and that occasional bowl of ice cream is less likely to sit on your waistline, thus avoiding the dreaded muffin top.

Another adaptation is the body making more mitochondria per each muscle cell, creating efficient use of the fuel in your body. This also increases the amount of enzymes that break down glucose and fat, resulting in a quicker response time for the body to produce the needed energy when movement of the body is required. This type of quick movement can be very important when one is required to move quickly such as when grabbing a child before they walk into a busy street. Eventually, muscle fibers will increase in size and number to assist in a more fuel efficient body, ultimately making exercising at higher intensities feel easier.

As you age, there is more fat stored in between the muscle fibers, which shows up in an X-ray as big white patches. This adaptation occurs in sedentary people as a way of protecting the body from severe muscle shrinkage. Permanent loss of muscle, or Sarcopenia, creates a mechanical issue of what material will make up the muscle to maintain muscle volume as this volume is essential to a healthy design. It is like trying to decide what material to use to finish a concrete slab if concrete is no longer available. Dirt or wood can be used, but neither material will create a strong, long-lasting foundation. Our bodies need to fill in the spaces in between muscle fibers and if it is not muscle, then the default material is fat. This excess intramuscular (inside the muscle) fat is not a good thing, as it doesn't contribute to a healthy retirement plan. It is not the healthy, functional muscle that will be needed as we age. Conversely, the muscles of a fit individual have less fat stored in them, and the muscle mass consists of actual muscle. Since muscle is the place where fuel is burned for energy – you do not burn calories in your fat cells – the best weight control program is to maintain a large amount of muscle and to keep it aerobically fit.

BENEFITS OF CARDIOVASCULAR FITNESS

Benefits of increased cardiovascular fitness are even more numerous than you think. Your heart will work efficiently and be less prone to disease. You will sleep better. Your mood and outlook will improve. Your brain will work better. Aerobic exercise is also the most effective non-pharmacological therapy for depression, especially in older adults. Research has shown that even when individuals require medication for depression, exercise has a beneficial effect. There is no known cap on the amount of aerobic exercise and its positive effects with regards to depression. In other words, the more spin classes you take, the better. Many patients with depression are able to reduce the dose of prescribed medications, and in some cases, they can stop taking them completely when they engage in a regular endurance exercise program.

The mood altering effects of exercise are often overlooked as many North Americans resort to prescribed anti-depressants and anti-anxiety medications. Valium, a well-known anti-anxiety medication, has the honor of being the biggest selling drug in the history of medicine. The increase in anxiety disorders can be correlated to an increasingly sedentary population and easy access to poor food that is not only unhealthy but addictive.

Another benefit of aerobic exercise is that it can almost always be done as a social activity. In this crazy, busy world in which socializing can be so difficult and no one has time to just hang out, choosing to exercise in groups or with a buddy can lead to the creation of strong social connections. Building and maintaining friendships has all kinds of positive effects on health, from reducing the risk factors for heart disease to increasing memory and cognitive function. In the spring and summer in Victoria BC, it is commonplace to see cyclists out enjoying a group ride together. I remember riding my bike into Victoria from Salt Spring when a cycling group passed by me. Several members of the group spoke to me for a few moments, and I learned that they were a (men's only) group that rode together once a week as they all smiled and chatted with energy and enthusiasm. The men in this group were of all ages and fitness levels, out together and enjoying the companionship as much as the exercise.

Even when going through a rough patch in my life, I continued to exercise and join friends for regular hiking and cycling and found the consistent companionship helped get me through it. These days, I attend a Bellyfit class twice a week on Salt Spring, and every time I arrive, my instructor Trina Aspinall greets me with a hug and enthusiasm as we catch up on family, life, and local happenings.

THE NUMBER ONE KILLER: HEART DISEASE

Heart disease is the leading cause of death in North America, killing more people every year than the four other leading causes of death (cancer, chronic lower respiratory disease, accidents and stroke). High blood pressure, high cholesterol, obesity, and diabetes are all risk factors for heart disease. Once a person has heart disease, they are at high risk of experiencing heart failure. Heart attacks are the leading cause of death amongst adults in the developed world. Recently, studies have shown a 46 percent reduction in the risk of heart failure by engaging daily in one hour of moderate aerobic exercise or 30 minutes of more intense aerobic exercise.

High blood pressure is a risk factor for many fatal diseases like heart attacks and strokes. One in three adults in North America suffers from high blood pressure that is straining their blood vessel walls. Obesity is a risk factor for developing high blood pressure, but even small changes in an individual's weight can increase blood pressure. Notable studies have demonstrated that as little as five to 11 pounds of weight gain can force the blood pressure up. Consider how many of us have experienced weight gain after going away for a weekend getaway or lengthy holiday. Engaging in a regular aerobics exercise program where the heart rate is up and the sweat is flowing will reduce blood pressure, lower cholesterol, and increase insulin sensitivity. The exercise itself has a direct effect on risk factors, but the secondary effects of exercise, such as weight loss, improved body composition, better sleep, and improved mood are equally as important.

Your heart and lungs are made up of muscle fibers, and it is often overlooked that they, too, need to be exercised just like other muscle tissue. Just like a leg or arm muscle, the heart and lung muscles need to be considered in the design of an exercise program. In a de-conditioned individual, it takes time for the heart and lungs to function in an efficient manner. Quite often, the burning that we feel in our chest and throat as we get our heart rate up is the lung muscle trying to get caught up to meet the demands of the rest of the body. The heart muscle needs time to become conditioned to be able to work hard enough to pump blood more efficiently throughout the body. If you have any diseases of the heart or lungs, consider this before starting a cardiovascular conditioning exercise program. This does not mean that you should not engage in an aerobic exercise program as studies are revealing the benefits of aerobic exercise even after a heart attack or stroke or after being diagnosed with a lung disease. As your heart and lung muscles adapt, exercise will seem easier, making the process more enjoyable.

There are many different ways to become aerobically fit. The most important thing is to find something that you enjoy and to mix up your activities to avoid boredom and overuse injuries. I recently came across a report from York University's School of Health in Toronto that suggested that people think they are exercising more intensely than they actually are. I used to see this in my gym amongst my members and clients. Many people do not train long enough during their exercise sessions, or at high enough intensities to produce the metabolic effects of endurance training. It is critical to work out at certain intensities to achieve those physiological changes right down at the cellular level.

Once you become aerobically fit – the definition of this depends on your age, health status, and goals – then it becomes a matter of maintenance. Unless you have a disease or condition that prevents you from exercising at higher intensities, high-intensity training (HIT) should become part of your weekly routine. HIT has become all the rage in the fitness industry over the last few years because you burn a total of more calories during an HIT session, and you get aerobically fit faster, which creates a physiological environment to burn more calories after your exercise sessions.

There are a few factors that need to be considered before jumping into an HIT program. The fact that your ligaments, tendons, and muscles will be at a higher risk for injury unless they are properly conditioned for a more vigorous exercise program should be considered, as well as; your age and health status, and your willingness to work at high intensities. If sprinting up one flight of stairs could permanently turn you off from exercising, then HIT may not be for you. However, there are many benefits to exercising at higher intensities. Women will be interested to know that getting really hot and sweaty is extremely beneficial after menopause. It was not very long ago that sweating was only considered polite for horses but certainly not for women. Kudos to the modern world where we get to feel and look as good as we choose.

PRACTICE MAKES PERFECT. PATIENCE IS NEEDED

Severely de-conditioned individuals will make progress with just a minimal amount of exercise during the first few months. But after the first few months, a plan needs to be in place for achieving enough exercise time to continue getting results. The recommended amount of weekly exercise, particularly after the age of fifty, is six hours, which includes two hours of weight resistant training and four hours of cardiovascular training, with some of that cardio training time at higher intensities. Yes, higher intensity translates into the sweating, red faced, maximal effort of an individual working really hard. If getting to the sweaty, red-faced phase is difficult to face, a good solution is to purchase a heart rate monitor and consult a fitness professional regarding the best heart rate and duration for your age and health status. Trust me, it will be time and money well spent.

The key thing to remember is that if you have a plan and stick to it, the results will speak for themselves. As discussed in a previous chapter, keep a journal and write down the hours of exercise that you are collecting each week. At the same time, make notes about how hard you worked during each exercise session.

Plan ahead for the week and make sure you create opportunities for a more intense workout. Hike up a steep hill for 60 minutes without stopping. Take a friend and race them to the top. Ride your bike on challenging routes and – don't avoid the hills. Take a spin class or two or find a dance class to attend. Play pick-up sports with friends or your kids or try out a boot camp class or Cross Fit class. Depending on the climate in your area, you can choose different seasonal activities throughout the year such as skiing in the winter and hiking in the summer. Whatever you choose, look at it as an opportunity for fun and adventure.

Choice of the activity matters as there are healing sports and then other sports that can, over the long term, cause the breakdown of your joints. For example, continued running on concrete can lead to arthritic changes in your knees and hips, and racquet sports like tennis can cause similar damage to your joints. Swimming, cycling, and cross-country skiing, on the other hand, are considered healing sports as they are much easier on the joints. I have found that cross-training is very important in preventing injuries, arthritis, and chronic joint issues. If you play soccer, basketball, or baseball, you can balance your exercise plan with a weekly swim. Adding a trail run to your weekly running schedule can reduce the effects of the impact of road running. Balancing out downhill skiing with cross-country skiing has benefits like maintaining interest and enthusiasm for exercising while reducing potential injuries. Learning a new skill is good for the brain and for the body, so if you love to play tennis why not take up swimming? Swimming is something you can do on your off days to recover without losing aerobic fitness.

There are so many aerobic activities to choose from once you get started. Not only will you begin to feel and look better, but you will also meet some very interesting people along the way. Lifetime friendships and partnerships happen when you get out and try new activities. Muscles are the machine and cardio fitness is the fuel that will let that machine move without running out of gas.

7:

The Zen of the Treadmill

When I moved to Salt Spring Island in 1998, I was looking for a different lifestyle. My first marriage had ended, partly as a result of my rebellion against being in a traditional, patriarchal relationship and partly due to my desire to explore a healthier lifestyle. Landing on Salt Spring in the middle of summer was a dreamy experience. I witnessed a combination of beauty and grace, unlike anything I had ever experienced. The island's magic wrapped itself around my heart and gently pulled me into the expanse of its loving warmth, leaving me wanting more.

My second visit to the island resulted in me purchasing a house and arranging to move my tribe of five children to Salt Spring before the start of the new school year. Of all the decisions I have ever made, the one to move to sleepy Salt Spring Island changed everything. Every belief, every habit, every thought was shaken and turned upside down the very moment I stepped off that ferry, all those years ago. Until that moment, I had been like many others. I kept my head down, forged ahead and didn't question anything. I just moved one foot forward and never looked up to see what direction I was going in.

After the move, I began the slow, sometimes painful, sometimes joyful journey of reflection, awareness, and healing, which was, for me, all part of being quiet, being in nature, and being surrounded by others on a similar path. I learned that a soul's journey is meant to continue until, eventually, we die. Even the aboriginals in this area understood that the island is a place to heal in all ways.

After the first few years working as a personal trainer, I quickly realized that my clients needed not only to regularly exercise their bodies but also to regularly turn off their minds, at least for a short time. Salt Spring is a haven for those seeking conscious wellness. Its majestic beauty, peace, and serenity are conducive to meditation, and meditation is instrumental in increasing awareness and self-exploration.

My friend, fellow author, and island resident John Cowhig practices Transcendental Meditation, about which he says the following:

"It is a simple technique that allows the mind to settle down through quieter and quieter levels of thought, until thought is transcended, and what remains is what we are: consciousness, being, pure awareness. Consciousness, being, is not only our essential nature, it's also the source of all energy, intelligence, and creativity, so connecting regularly means we begin to unfold our full potential, which is really, ultimately, cosmic. All possibilities are achievable with a human body and nervous system."

Meditation

The technique of Transcendental Meditation, as well as other styles of meditation, is becoming more understood and accepted by the general public. I decided to find a technique to help my clients incorporate the benefits of mindful practice with exercise, but in place of sitting cross-legged, I get them to hop on the treadmill.

Over the past twenty years, the study of neuropsychology has transformed as research continues to reveal that meditation works to relax both our minds and our bodies. Meditation has been practiced by spiritual masters for almost as long as humans have existed, and science is now, finally, recognizing what spiritual leaders have always known: that there is a correlation between longevity and having a regular meditation ritual. Through meditation, we focus on compassion, love, peace, joy and harmony. In his best-selling book *Buddha's Brain* (2009), Dr. Rick Hanson explains in simple terms how our brains function and how meditation can ease our suffering. Our minds are hardwired to suffer, to eat fat, and to be sedentary. There are very good scientific explanations for humans being attracted to these seemingly unhealthy conditions. Living in a condition where we are prone to suffering – consuming high-fat foods while rarely having the desire to get off the couch – sounds like the perfect material for a country and western song. I can hear it now: *Well the dog died, I lost my job, and my wife left. Just took right off with the keys and the car and I need a beer - but that dang beer fridge is so far away.*

What is the answer to this human condition? Meditation has the power to change our brains over time and it sure beats other methods that are used to *numb out*. It can get us out of those ruts that our over-thinking creates, partially because it requires sitting and focusing on breathing for extended periods of time in a quiet setting away from noise and distractions.

One of my former, and favorite, clients used to work for a large oil company based in Alberta, in what he described as "definitely a corporate world." He explained to me how someone in human resources decided that the employees should attend a meditation seminar. With the usual grumblings about a new workshop promoted by HR, the whole company gathered in a large hotel conference room.

As the group entered, they were instructed to sit on the floor, either cross-legged or in some variation of that position. As they all wrestled their stiff legs into unfamiliar contortions, no doubt missing the chairs, stage and podium of their usual staff meetings, the facilitator instructed the participants to sit quietly with their eyes closed and to focus on their breathing. According to my former client, the most amazing thing happened in that room. He said that after ten minutes of sitting still in absolute silence, several of his colleagues began to cry, finding themselves overwhelmed by being alone with their thoughts. This incident had a powerful effect on my client, inspiring him to begin meditating every day for at least half an hour.

My client is not alone. – Even Jack Canfield, the creator of the best-selling *Chicken Soup for the Soul* series, promotes the concept of the hour of power: twenty minutes of reading, twenty minutes of meditation, and twenty minutes of exercise every day. As it happens, twenty minutes of exercise a day translates into 140 minutes per week, which is close to the 150 minutes per week of moderate-intensity exercise recommended in the 2008 *Physical Activity Guidelines for Americans.*

Meditation has also been shown to reduce blood pressure and help to reduce pain from chronic inflammatory conditions like rheumatoid arthritis and muscular-skeletal pain syndromes. However, it is not easy to incorporate a regular practice of meditation into an already busy and often hectic life. If adding more to your plate causes stress, the benefits of the added activity will quickly be minimized. That is why I came up with a solution for the busy person who needs to exercise regularly and meditate for overall wellness. The solution to a lack of time and difficulty locating a dedicated space at home lies in getting to the gym.

The Treadmill

The treadmill is one of the finest inventions in the fitness industry. It does not take up much space. Its use is not dependent on the weather and conditions are always comfortable, though maybe a little warm once you get going. Most treadmills are designed with a soft deck that absorbs shock, making it much easier on your joints than running on hard surfaces. They are equipped with safety features like side bars, front handles, and a safety cord that shuts off the treadmill automatically to attach to your workout clothes in case you trip or fall while exercising. There is often a TV mounted to the front of the treadmill, as well as an iPod charger and headset plug, which means you can listen to your music without draining your device's battery.

Treadmills provide important information for the user such as the measurement of time, distance, pace, heart rate, and calories burned. There are different programs to choose from, for which the machine will simulate a course. For example, a user could select a 5km trail run, complete with hills and flat stretches. Treadmills can also be set at different inclines to increase the difficulty and to work different leg muscles.

Even though treadmills have been around for a long time, and other types of cardio equipment are continually being designed, treadmills still remain at the top of the list as the most popular piece of equipment at the gym.

Many people purchase treadmills to use at home, but real estate agents will tell you that the number-one use of a home treadmill is for hanging laundry. One should consider this fact carefully before making the investment. Another consideration in the home-versus-gym conundrum is quality. Most commercial treadmills are close to ten thousand dollars each. They are solidly built and include many extras both to appeal to a wide range of customers and withstand years of pounding. The home versions cost considerably less, but they do not have the same quality as the commercial variety. The difference is comparable to driving a cheap little car without any options when you could have access to a sleeker more luxurious vehicle with all the bells and whistles.

Back to the Zen part of this chapter. Your gym will offer a lineup of treadmills so make sure you choose your favorite machine, in your favorite spot. Place your sweat towel over the front of the TV to stop you from getting distracted by the screen. During meditation, you won't be watching TV! However, it is a good idea to bring an iPod or another device to listen to your preferred meditation music or guided meditation that will drown out the gym noise and help you to get into the zone. If you are new to the Zen of the Treadmill program, progress slowly. It is suggested to start with five minutes at a time and progress up to 30 minutes per session. Remember, the goal here is twofold: to quiet your mind and to get some exercise.

You have secured your favorite treadmill, your headphones are in place, your sweat towel is ready and you've placed your water bottle in the holder. Now it's time to get going. Start with a few minutes of walking to warm up. Once you are feeling warm and relaxed, you can begin your meditation practice. When a thought pops into your head, take a brief moment to observe that thought and let it go. Focusing on your breathing will make it possible to stop focusing on your thoughts. This process takes time and patience, which is why you start slowly and work up to thirty minutes.

While you are walking or jogging on the treadmill, distractions will pop into your vision range and mind. You'll notice and become curious about the man at the other end of the gym who is trying to bench press 400 pounds. When you notice, stop and let it go! The woman wearing really tight neon colors may catch your eye. Stop and let it go! You suddenly remember that your boss needs that report early the next morning so why are you even at the gym instead of at the office working! Stop and let it go. Your head is buzzing with the fact that your mother-in-law is arriving tonight for two weeks. Yes, even that—just stop and let it go! You're worried that your teenage daughter is spending too much time alone with her boyfriend. Stop and let it go! Your left calf muscle is talking to you and it's going to cramp. Stop and let it go! This is getting tedious. Just stop and let it go!

Pretty soon you will be able to last for thirty minutes in a state of peace and quiet. Thoughts will come and go, but you will not focus on any of them. All of a sudden, when you finish thirty minutes on the treadmill, you realize that the time passed without discomfort. Your thoughts are not controlling you and you have just worked off three hundred calories. After a few months of this program, you will look forward to your treadmill time. Your clothes will fit better and your head won't feel dangerously close to exploding on a regular basis. You've found a solution that's better than drugs and alcohol and is far less expensive. Instead of beer bottles floating in your head, you see treadmills in your daydreams. This is the true Zen of the Treadmill. You have achieved an altered state, with a short trip to your favorite treadmill at your favorite club, your heart is open, your mind is free, and your muscles are exercised. Does it get any better?

8:

Move Over Big Pharma—Now is the Age of Preventative Medicine

There is a silent storm occurring silently throughout North America. With media focusing on environmental issues, climate change, and the threat of terrorist attacks, there is little discussion about the pharmaceutical industry. Unfortunately, most of us are susceptible to the mass media's hype, finding ourselves guilty of enjoying the gossipier, sensationalistic stories than the practical, less exciting information. True, news reports about an aging population and subsequent health issues are not exactly sexy or mediagenic. The pharmaceutical industry and its effects are not particularly sexy or sensationalistic either, nor do they create mass fear or hysteria like stories of an Ebola outbreak in the United States. However, this book is about the future of fitness and the benefits of joining a gym. The information presented in this book may not be particularly mediagenic, but it is thought provoking and essential for a transition towards a more prevention-based health care model. In any case, a discussion about future change cannot take place without a conversation about the medical establishment generally and the pharmaceutical industry specifically.

In 2012, the pharmaceutical industry in Canada reported sales of $21.6 billion. (In the States, prescription drug sales are reported to be over a trillion dollars.) Canada's pharmaceutical sales have nearly doubled in just over a decade, up from $11.7 billion dollars in 2001. The top five selling drugs are as follows: Remicade, an anti-arthritic medication; Crestor, a cholesterol-lowering agent; Humira, another anti-arthritic medication; Enbrel, yet another anti-arthritic medication; and Lucentis, which is for vision loss. The pharmaceutical industry in Canada employed 23,468 people in 2001 and 26,945 people by 2013.

In contrast, let's look at the fitness industry. In 2013, the fitness industry in Canada was a two-billion-dollar industry with over 4500 fitness clubs across the country employing 47,957 people. Just over 15 percent of Canadians are members of a gym. The fitness industry has not doubled in the last ten years, but it *should* have doubled because apparently, based on the above pharmaceutical statistics, the general population is suffering from an epidemic of arthritis, and exercise is a major player in both prevention and treatment of arthritis. As mentioned above, three out of the five top-selling medications in Canada are for arthritis, with annual sales of over $1.2 billion. That would indicate that prescriptions for arthritis are greater than 6 percent of the total sales of all pharmaceuticals in Canada. As a matter of fact, the top ten drugs sold in Canada were for diseases and conditions that are positively affected by exercise and nutrition. These include drugs to reduce cholesterol, reduce arthritic pain, to deal with depression, for stomach acid control, and for asthma.

The other critical issue that is overlooked is the total number of jobs created in the fitness industry versus the pharmaceutical industry. Let's take a closer look at the statistics. The pharmaceutical industry employs 26,945 people, whereas the fitness industry employees 47,957 people, but the fitness industry is only a two-billion-dollar a year industry while the pharmaceutical industry is worth over $21 billion a year. In spite of the difference in total sales, the fitness industry employs almost twice as many people as the pharmaceutical industry. This contrast in numbers is significant. When I was at university in the 1980s, I took a course in natural resource economics, and during the course, the professor talked about the social net benefit versus social cost of different industries. Using this principle to review the fitness industry, it could be stated that the social net benefit of the fitness sector far outweighs the cost to society. Furthermore, as the fitness industry grows, the benefit to society will grow exponentially, especially if you factor in job creation. On the other hand, the social net benefit of the pharmaceutical industry is diminished by the cost. These costs will be discussed in more detail throughout this chapter. From the absolute numbers alone, we see from the above statistics that as the pharmaceutical industry expands, the relative number of employment opportunities does not keep pace. The lack of relative employment is a loss to society, even before taking into account the environmental pollution caused by manufacturing drugs and the side effects associated with the consumption of pharmaceuticals.

HOW DID BIG PHARMA GET SO BIG?

The first question is how did this rapid increase in pharmaceutical sales happen? The answer is not simple, and demographics can only explain part of the increase in drug sales, particularly anti-arthritic medications. As the population ages, certain medical conditions increase, often due to the sedentary lifestyle of most Canadians. Prepackaged and poor quality food has led to many health challenges that eventually cause a trip to the doctor's office for a visit and a prescription.

How doctors are reimbursed has an effect. Doctors are paid on a per patient visit so naturally they tend to keep the appointments short, leaving little time for explaining alternatives to drugs or counseling about lifestyle changes. Then there is the matter of patient compliance to consider. If a doctor spends his or her time discussing lifestyle changes and the patient does not comply and their symptoms get worse, the doctor is held responsible. Patient compliance is very low, and family doctors are aware of this. I realized very early on as a personal trainer that what people hear from their medical professional and what was actually said are two different things. Often, when my clients described what advice they had been given from their healthcare practitioner, it was obvious that there was a problem in communication. A person who is in pain or anxious about their health can easily misunderstand information, especially if they don't take notes or if the appointment is rushed. In the end, a prescription is written because it is easy to do and the result is richer drug companies while fitness levels decrease.

The next question is why isn't the fitness industry keeping a similar pace to big pharma? There are some obvious reasons for this. Every year *Maclean's* magazine publishes the top ten industries that lobby the federal government. Pharmaceutical companies are routinely listed in the top ten, but nowhere on this list is the fitness industry represented. In spite of the social net benefit to society and the number of jobs that this industry creates, the money in the fitness business does not equal the money that drugs generate. And as we all know, politicians are busy and don't always have an understanding of health issues or the science behind alternatives to pharmaceuticals.

In order to promote health and its positive effects, an effort will have to be made to focus on both funding and policies to support industries that offer job creation, minimal environmental impact, and overall healthier communities. Just like environmentalists look toward alternative energy sources to reduce greenhouse gasses, I am suggesting that we look toward the fitness industry to reduce health care costs and to slow down the runaway train of pharmaceutical sales.

CASE STUDY ONE: ADULT ONSET DIABETES

A good example of fitness professionals coming together with doctors in a team approach to look for solutions outside of surgery and using prescription drugs is in the treatment of type 2 diabetes, also known as adult onset diabetes. This type of diabetes is not to be confused with type 1 diabetes, which occurs when the pancreas quits producing insulin altogether. In the case of type 2 diabetes, the receptors on the cell membranes lose sensitivity and efficiency. Insulin is needed to carry glucose (sugar in its simplest form) through the cell membrane into the cell to be used as fuel for the muscles. If the cell membrane is no longer sensitive to insulin, glucose is unable to enter the cell and the levels of glucose in the blood-stream begin to rise.

Among other health risks, chronically elevated blood sugar levels can cause damage to the eyes, increase the risk of infections, increase the risk of heart disease and cause weight gain. Currently, prescription pills for adult onset diabetes may make blood sugar results look better, but they don't actually improve the function of the body to optimal health. These drugs do not restore normal cellular function, do not give the patient a nourishing diet, nor do they educate the patient about the importance of a smart and effective exercise program. A "smart" exercise program simply means that exercise training is specifically designed for a certain health condition.

Adult onset diabetes is the result of a lengthy progression of metabolic changes in which your genes play only a minor role, meaning the condition is not genetic. The factors within your control that are leading causes of adult onset diabetes are physical inactivity, unmanaged stress, poor nutrient intake, and inadequate sleep. Beyond managing these factors, a patient needs to work with their doctor. The doctor does not need to be involved with the "smart exercise" program except to refer the patient to a personal trainer, who can engage their client in a successful exercise regime. In my opinion, a family doctor should recommend more than just moving regularly. He or she should prescribe "smart exercise" and recommend a trip to the gym to enlist the support of a personal trainer.

Smart exercise refers to choosing the method of exercise known to help with a specific disease like adult onset diabetes. A certified personal trainer is educated about exercise prescription and understands what exercises are the greatest benefit and the least risk to their clients. With adult-onset diabetes, it is highly recommended to lift heavier weights with fewer repetitions than engaging only in light aerobic training.

In our gym, we had many people present with high blood sugar. Mostly they were on medication and were not aware of the benefits of weight lifting. Once these clients went through a vigorous weight lifting program, they were able to reduce their dependence on medication or get off their meds completely. It was a tremendous relief both emotionally and financially to our clients to get fitter and less dependent on prescription medication. I can still remember clients grinning from ear to ear as they announced that they had been given the all-clear to stop taking medicine to reduce their blood sugar. It was like they had come home with an A on their report card, proudly handing it over to a happy parent. (Except, in this case, we, as the trainers, were the proud parents.)

This is a great example of a team effort between a health care professional and professional fitness trainer. With adult onset diabetes, drugs are meant for worst-case scenarios, not as the first line of defense. The future looks good in this new strategy of collaboration with a team that accepts that a patient can take charge of their own health, and where no one on the team gives up.

CASE STUDY TWO: ARTHRITIS

The next example is arthritis, a condition which, given the sales of anti-arthritic medication, appears to be epidemic in Canada. Arthritis is understood by the general public to be a painful condition that affects various joints in the body. As with any structural design, there are places of weakness in the body. There are elements of the structure that are more likely to collapse under a load. Our joints are places where wear and tear are most likely to occur, and the two joints that are the most susceptible are the hip and the knee joints.

After fifteen years of working as a personal trainer with thousands of bodies – some of those bodies for many years – I am aware of patterns of dysfunction in the joints. The gradual breakdown of joints happens over years, causing problems well before the pain symptoms begin. Arthritis occurs primarily because of muscle imbalances. These imbalances are a result of poor posture, overuse injuries, and/or stress. Our sedentary culture has created most of our postural imbalances, and when you combine that with poor nutrition, obesity, limited exercise, and chronic stress, you have a recipe for disaster.

Only in the last fifteen to twenty years has posture been recognized as a major contributor to joint and muscle pain. There are many treatment modalities for arthritis and muscular pain, other than reaching for a pill bottle. I feel very strongly that anyone suffering from any kind of muscular or joint pain at any age should be sent by their physician to see a fitness professional to look at posture and lifestyle. This would help prevent so much of the misery that people suffer later on in their life as arthritis sets in.

A common myth around arthritis is that exercise makes the joints worse. There is a perception that joint pain and swelling will be aggravated by exercise. The whole understanding of this disease is complicated because people assume that any joint pain they have is arthritis and that arthritis is part of the normal aging process. The beliefs that people have about pain create a defeatist attitude that is also promoted by the marketing of both over-the-counter and prescription painkillers by drug sales reps to doctors. There was a very interesting study that was published in the *New England Journal of Medicine* in 2002 on the placebo effect of surgery on patients with debilitating knee pain. There were three groups of individuals in this study. Two of the groups had standard practice surgery for arthritic knees, and the third group, being the placebo group, went through the pretense of surgery, including three standard incisions.

All three groups were sent to rehab and given specific rehabilitation exercises. The results of the study were astounding. The placebo group improved as much as the two surgery groups. There were follow-up videos taken of people walking and playing basketball from the placebo group; activities that they could not do before the surgery. The placebo group did not find out that they had not actually had real surgery until two years after the study. This is a telling example of how our beliefs impact our reality.

The trainers at my gym would take a client with pain in their joints and put them on a rehab program to start, treating these clients as if they had just had surgery, reassuring them that they would be fine. This approach worked, and we witnessed amazing results. When I read about the study mentioned above, I wondered how much of the improvement from surgery, or perceived surgery, was a result of the follow-up, rehabilitative exercise program.

The interesting thing about pain is that it is the body's only way of sending a message to the brain that something is wrong. There needs to be a new paradigm about pain instilled in people's minds to move away from instantly reaching for those painkillers. Muscles hold our joints together so they can function optimally with minimal wear and tear. If our muscles are not working properly or are weak from inactivity, then wear and tear of joints is on speed dial. As soon as an individual begins to experience pain, either in their joints or muscles, it is time to turn to a team of experts to get assistance in realigning the body's structure. This team needs to include a family doctor, a qualified physiotherapist, a massage therapist, and a fitness expert at your gym who can design a complete exercise program tailored to your individual needs.

Taking painkillers will provide temporary pain relief and are clearly necessary for acute pain situations such as recovery from surgery or an accident, but they are deadly for chronic pain or pain as a result of lifestyle choices or poor posture. Medication masks pain but the conditions for wear and tear remain unchanged. The side effects of ingestion of painkillers are relevant, and eventually, the body will send increasingly severe pain signals until even the strongest meds stop working. At this point surgery is usually the only recourse.

If anyone who is reading this chapter has ever needed joint replacement surgery, they can attest to the debilitating pain they suffered while they waited for their turn on the operating table. Even if surgery is the only option, it is imperative to keep moving. Post-surgery rehab is essential to get back normal function of the muscles around a surgically replaced joint. There are many exercises that can be engaged in at the gym no matter where you are in the pre- and post-surgery spectrum. Sometimes injury and/or surgery can be an opportunity to discover the benefits of exercise and become educated about exercise selection and the benefits of improved posture. Reaching for the gym bag will be the new prescription for joint pain as doctors and the general public recognize the freedom in pain relief by natural methods.

Fitness in the future must involve collaboration between doctors and fitness professionals. I believe that, through government policies and education, the use of pharmaceuticals will begin to slow down and exercise will be prescribed as often as medications. As a result, the overall health of communities will improve and enjoyment of life will increase. No disease is a result of a drug deficiency. Pharmaceuticals will always have their place, but not as big of a place, as we become what we were always meant to be: fit and healthy.

9:

Make 60 the New 40

If you have never had a fitness trainer as your friend, you have no idea what you are missing. My friends and clients have told me that surely my true calling was to be a drill sergeant, but through a strange twist of fate, I became a personal trainer instead. Every time I take a personality test, I never seem to score high in the soft, cuddly, or nurturing category. Phrases such as *has trouble listening, takes charge* and *wants to give direction* are more along the lines of my test results. Luckily, in my profession, if you take charge and give clear directions without listening to complaints, you end up providing a good workout for your clients.

Including a fitness trainer in your circle of friends will also alter your beliefs, especially your perceptions about aging. Most of the population unconsciously assumes that one simply gets old and then dies. This is a belief whose power can, and does, have negative consequences, and is no way to plan for your golden years. Unlike the average person, fitness trainers have a vision of life that includes the possibility of life being active and exciting up until the very end.

My friend Janine is an example of someone whose life has been affected by having a close friendship with a personal trainer – me. Statistically speaking, Janine is an average woman in many ways. She is in her mid-50s, average height, weight, and dress size. However, she consistently proves to be above average as a friend. Janine was raised in a typical middle class, hard-working Canadian family. I met Janine when I first opened my membership gym, and she soon became a client and a friend. We had an instant connection when we first met. Janine is both witty and charming, interested in staying in shape, and enjoying life. When we realized that Janine's babysitter, when she was really young, was my former husband's oldest sister in a small farming town in Alberta, we knew we were destined to be friends.

Back when we first met, Janine was struggling with the typical issues of the middle-aged. She was adjusting to changing hormone levels, keeping the body fat at bay, and dealing with graying hair. For most in their late forties, job stress is high, parents are aging, and the kids are hitting the hellish teen years. This age group is caring both for their parents and their children, and therefore, it is often called the sandwich generation.

These years are also the years in which anxiety around sex and drugs with teenage children either destroys your own sex life, or has you – and not the teenager – reaching for the calming effects of drugs. Janine does not have children, but she has witnessed enough teenage angst vicariously, through myself and other friends, to know that it is a tough stage for any parent to deal with.

Janine first sought my expertise to deal with several pain syndromes that were just beginning, and she was feeling her energy and enthusiasm beginning to slow down. Her naturopath prescribed a visit to my gym to have an assessment and get started on a proper exercise program. Janine had been going to another gym regularly but seemed to have hit a plateau. Because Janine and I are close in age, and because she is clever, she did not bother with the "Well, you are younger and therefore don't understand" statement that is often used by clients as a justification for not taking my advice. Janine started a fairly rigorous exercise program under my supervision and with the support of my friendship. Soon, many of her aches and pains disappeared.

My beliefs about aging are very different than most of my contemporaries. I believe you can do anything you want, as long as you keep challenging yourself. A universal truth is that we are meant to fully enjoy our lives, to continue to be healthy, fit, and capable up until the end. It has never made sense to me to give energy into beliefs that ultimately reduce a person's ability to live fully and completely.

Janine did not buy into the 'getting old and dying' mentality, but she was concerned about losing her youthful energy and zest for life. The more time we spend together, the more I can see her desire to remain 40 as she heads for 60. Janine's attention to her hair, skin, and clothes are a huge part of her staying forty-something. Janine regularly gets her hair stylishly cut and colored, she uses good skincare products, and she does not smoke or drink. Because she looks after herself and has the desire to get out and socialize, my family considers Janine to be in a neutral age category. With an ageless ease and grace, she fits into any situation.

The true effect of her attitude was obvious when I decided to become familiar with TRX training. I invited Janine to be one of the guinea pigs as I tried out the TRX routine on a few clients. The most challenging exercise in the routine is to place one foot in a strap that is attached to the top of a door or post. Then you put your hands on the ground and lift your free leg straight up in the air so, effectively, you are in a handstand. Then you do pushups – yes, pushups – with the blood rushing to your head, your shoulders screaming, and all the while making sure that your legs don't move.

Janine looked at me with raised eyebrows as I demonstrated the exercise. I then helped her into the correct position and told her to lift her leg up. With her arms shaking like leaves on a tree on a windy day, she held the position for about five seconds. After I helped her get back on her feet, shaking and red in the face, she admitted that she had never done a handstand, headstand, or cartwheel, even when she was a child. It was an amazing moment for both of us. Janine had the belief that she could do it, she wanted to do it, and she didn't give up, and as her trainer, I knew it would be an extreme challenge for her, but did not want to hold her back by suggesting that she wasn't capable. After all, no one can do handstands unless they practice doing handstands.

How impossible is it in your head to do really difficult physical feats? Janine has a very high impossibility ceiling, referring to the limits she thinks are possible for herself. Sure her arms were sore for a few days, but her sense of accomplishment more than made up for her tired muscles. Janine has always wanted to be fully engaged in life but realized that she needed to stretch her comfort zone regularly in order to keep that engagement. Janine understands that success lies just outside your comfort zone and hanging out with people who stretch your comfort levels and challenge your beliefs is all part of staying 40ish when you are closer to 60ish.

Many experts on aging believe that there will be an overwhelming paradigm shift, occurring over the next twenty years, which will lead us to understand that decay is optional. Individuals like Janine who start to experience slowing down need to understand on an intuitive level that it is not *natural*.

The same radical shift in philosophy will occur with respect to our acceptance of deterioration as an inevitable part of aging. We will no longer accept decay of the body, decay of the brain, and decay of our spirits as a rite of passage.

As the body slows down, there is an opportunity to become spiritually aware. This can be the perfect time to enjoy family and friends, mentor young people starting their careers, contribute as a volunteer, reflect on the meaning of life, and engage in creative leisure time projects. The way society has approached aging, through advertising and marketing, and keeping generations physically separated, has caused fear and misunderstanding of this beautiful time in the human experience.

The reality is that the average age of humans has been radically extended by health care and better living conditions. In Canada, the average life expectancy is 81.57 years for men and women combined. The median age is now 40.2, up from 28 in 1971, due to increased longevity and declining birth rates. Over the next 50 years, the percentage of the population over the age of 75 will go from 6.9 to 14.6, meaning there will be more people in the over 75 age group than in the 14 and under age group. This may be seen by some as a blessing and by others as a curse, but one thing is for sure, we all need to plan for it.

There is talk about longevity decreasing in the long run as a result of poor diet and lifestyle. I'd like to offer a reality check here. Understand that no matter what shape you are in, continued technological advancements are likely to keep you alive, regardless of your ability to enjoy life.

There is one pertinent issue about aging that needs to be considered, and that is the notion of early retirement. In his book *The Demographic Cliff: How to Survive and Prosper During the Great Deflation of 2014–2019* (2014), Harry S. Dent Jr. calls retirement "bullshit." He makes an argument that, financially, people cannot be supported for more than ten years past retirement. It is not sustainable to retire at 55 and collect retirement income for another 25 years or more, nor is it a good idea emotionally, as it is a fundamental need of humans to contribute to and be part of a social network.

My experience as a fitness trainer and gym owner taught me many valuable lessons about life. One of the most valuable was the realization that retirement is a bad idea. Retiring early, or retiring completely, is the biggest way to fast forward the aging process, and I was witness to this through my clients and people in my own family. I noticed that once my clients retired they became less inspired and motivated. Many seemed to be going through the motions of exercise and did not have any focus or goal. In comparison, those working or engaged in a project that had deadlines were forced to hustle and be in a routine. In spite of being forced to adhere to a set schedule, these clients were happy and always had something to talk about and look forward to. In my own family, those who retired gained weight, became sick, and generally withdrew from life. I remember my grandfather, who was a tall formidable man that worked in the financial sector for over 40 years, took to a wheelchair and died soon after retiring. Even as a young woman, I could see how much my grandfather missed feeling like he was part of a group and contributing to something larger than himself. It was like he shrunk physically and emotional as soon as his career ended. This is not uncommon for retirees who still have so much life to give and live.

An inspiring example of non-retirement is Tony, a man who came almost every day to the gym and worked out hard enough to sweat profusely. Tony had a few biomechanical issues that would deter most people from ever joining a gym, never mind attending regularly. Tony was well past retirement age, which I only discovered by looking at his paperwork. Simply observing him gave me no indication of his age.

When I first met Tony, he seemed to be in his late 50s, tall, handsome, and very charming. He had a big smile and lots of confidence - the kind of confidence a man has in his prime. He greeted me with a twinkle in his eye and even flirted with me, and it was hard to resist his charisma. Then, when I filled out his paperwork, I had to stop myself from blurting out, "You're kidding, I simply can't believe that you are older than my father."

When Tony first bought a gym membership and pool access card, he informed me that he could only buy three months at a time because he was going overseas to work for the UN in a developing country. He had retired and moved to Salt Spring Island but decided to go back to work because he had so much experience and expertise to offer. He had made up his mind to enjoy his last decades and recognized that his desire to continue working required a healthy body. This was a motivator to keep him working out regularly. Tony knew that the only thing that would stop him would be poor health or a poor attitude.

According to Harry S. Dent Jr., we will all be working until we are close to 75 as retirement age is slowly increased by government policy, but that will only be possible when people develop a habit of regular exercise.

The other consideration about the new longevity that is giving us another 20 to 30 years of living is the quality of life, as there is little doubt that we will enjoy quantity. If you reach your late 50s and have not suffered any serious health issues, the reality is that you will live for another 20 to 30 years. Spending ten years or more confined to a chair or a walker as a means of being mobile is not a great prospect, never mind the pain from osteoarthritis and other muscular pain syndromes related to poor posture and lifestyle choices.

Dr. Henry S. Lodge, co-author of *Younger Next Year* (2007) states that some 70 percent of premature deaths and premature aging is lifestyle related. Dr. Lodge claims that heart attacks, strokes, the common cancers, diabetes, brittle bones, most falls, fractures, and serious injuries are primarily caused by the way we live. We do have a choice in how we age. Create the new reality. Realize that, not only can we prevent illness and disease from prematurely taking away the joys of living, we can begin a glorious, active, and productive lifestyle that is indeed better than in earlier periods of our lives.

Think of all the amazing activities and extreme sports that seniors are engaging in and breaking the records in every day. There are 90-year-olds performing athletic feats that surpass the average 20-year-old. I regularly read posts on Facebook from *Growing Bolder* about the feats of the middle-aged and beyond. It is inspiring, to say the least, and changing our perception of what was once considered reality – the rocking chair on the porch – after middle age.

If we want to let our inner fitness freak fly, we need to embrace a new way of claiming life as we age and stay active and very fit. I am looking forward to joining all of those who embrace their freaky nature by taking on new adventures and possibly ending up myself on a poster on *Growing Bolder*.

So no more pictures of walkers and scooters in our heads! Instead, we should see images of 70 and 80-year-olds contributing to society. We should read stories about the older generation mentoring young people and remaining valued employees and employers. Age should be understood as the dawn of wisdom. My friend Janine understands how exercise will carry her forward into her third age, and Tony is living his dream of growing old with gladness. Both Janine and Tony have made the conscious choice to be producers and not prisoners of aging. We need our seniors, so please look after yourselves! My advice for the young is that they should plan and work towards beautiful and productive golden years.

10:
Community Matters

Salt Spring Island boasts some of the best running trails anywhere in North America. Not only are they beautiful and numerous, but they are also never crowded, even on the sunniest day. Today, I went off to run with the Salt Spring Trail Running group, a group that goes every Sunday morning, exploring a different route each week. There were over ten of us on this windy, sunny November day. It is unlikely that even half of the group would attempt such an outing without the companionship and support of the community of runners. As I ran through the beautiful woods, my thoughts turned to an article that was written by Dr. Walter Bortz, an American leader in advancing scientific principles of healthy aging. Check out his website for even more interesting stories and scientific research: http://www.walterbortz.com/ .

Dr. Bortz published an article on the first 100-year-old human (centenarian) to complete a marathon. The centurion, a man by the name of Fauja Singh, accomplished this feat at the Toronto Marathon in eight hours, twenty-five minutes, seventeen seconds. Singh took up marathon running at the age of 89 and is affectionately referred to by his close friends as the "turbaned tornado."

Running is a community sport, and even though some of us run alone to meditate and enjoy the solitude, all runners can appreciate the pleasure of the companionship of fellow joggers, – even if it is only at a running event. For large or small events, runners come together to feel a part of something bigger than themselves. How amazing it must have felt for Mr. Singh to be a part of that mass of energy and to finish the marathon with the crowd cheering him on! He inspired a throng of incredulous spectators to throw away their long-held beliefs about aging.

Connecting in the 21st Century

What is it that appeals to humans to participate in large athletic events? Tough Mudder is a great example of group participation. Imagine driving to the site of a Tough Mudder course and running the 20 km course by yourself, and braving the ice-cold pool where you have to swim under a board to get out, then run through two miles of mud up to your knee caps, get on your forearms and knees to crawl through mud without letting the barb-wire above you cut through your clothes. Then, just when you think it might end, you slide down an ice bank where the snow cuts your exposed skin just before you land in a lake half covered with ice. At the very end, when you are cold, muddy, hungry, and just plain grouchy, you run through wires and get shocked by many, and feel burns on your bare skin where you were electrocuted. This just for something to do – not bloody likely.

Whistler BC is home to an annual Tough Mudder event. Whistler, a world class ski resort and home of the 2010 Winter Olympic ski events, experiences its busiest day of the year, not on Christmas day, not on Boxing day or on New Year's Eve, but the Saturday in June when they hold Tough Mudder. On this day, over 20,000 crazy-ass people descend on Whistler Village to run through 20 km of mud, snow, cold water, and military-style obstacles.

In 2010, there were 200,000 participants in obstacle races in North America with $15.9 million in revenue. By 2014, there were over 4 million participants with $362 million in revenue. What is our fascination?

I participated in Tough Mudder two years in a row and witnessed teamwork and bonding as people worked together in overcoming difficult challenges, mimicking the cave man instinct that is still present in our DNA. This is a community. This is what it means to be human on the most basic level. As the "mudders" were helping each other over the obstacles, I could imagine a group hunt where everyone was needed for a successful kill. The survival of the tribe would have been dependent on keeping even the weakest member alive. Pre-agrarian conditions were so harsh that all babies that survived to adulthood were necessary to ensure the long-term survival of the group.

The most beautiful memory I have from my participation in Tough Mudder was watching a young woman in her early thirties struggle with every step to get to the top of a path built directly under the Olympic ski jump. The path was worn into a grassy bank and was almost vertical. This woman's teammates cheered and cheered and held out their arms to grab her as soon as she was close to the top. This challenge was at the end of the course and absolutely brutal, not only because it was incredibly slippery, but also because it was so steep that it caused calf and quad muscles to burn with every step. As this woman made two steps forward, she slid back a step.

I stopped to watch as her teammates grabbed her arms and pulled her to the flat spot at the top. They hugged her and each other and cheered as if someone had just finished a gold medal performance. I felt a lump in my throat and tears welled up, but it was more than simply teamwork that made me so emotional. It was a deep-seated need for everyone to be part of a group, to be included in a group, and to take care of the group members to ensure the survival of the tribe. Fauja Singh may not have finished the marathon, and certainly the young woman would never have made it through the Tough Mudder obstacles, without the loving, encouraging support of fellow humans.

The Community Can Stay Connected Through Communication and Health

The loss of community is not happening in the younger generation. In fact, the greatest loss of community that has the most tragic consequences is taking place within the older generation. I attended a Rotary Club meeting about two years ago and gave a presentation called "A Healthy

Community." The average age of the audience was 70 years, and the only comment came from a man who argued that cell phone use by younger people was ruining the world. I explained that, in fact, social media creates community and provides a way for each member to stay connected and communicate almost instantly. It provides a sense of belonging, not just to family and friends, but to the greater global community as well. Never before in the history of humankind have we been able to receive information instantly or have access to different sources of information and different ideas about what that information means.

Social Isolation causes a loss to the community, and the impact of that loss is most prevalent in our senior demographic and is not instigated by the use of cell phones by younger people. In fact, the cell phone creates a connection. If that man who commented to me at the Rotary Club meeting continues to live out his narrow view of the world, he could find himself becoming part of the tragedy of aging poorly like many of his contemporaries.

The generation of people 65 and older is the fastest growing demographic in Canada and many in this cohort are not aging well. There are health issues in this group directly related to lack of exercise, poor nutrition, and social isolation. The best place to read about these issues is *The State of Public Health in Canada 2014*. This report was compiled by the Chief Public Health Officer, Dr. Gregory Taylor, and is very well written and rich in content. Dr. Taylor summarizes his report by saying, "If the future is all about change, then we need to be the change that sets the future."

CHANGES THAT ARE HAPPENING AND HOW
COMMUNITIES CAN PLAN FOR THESE CHANGES

First of all, people living longer is just beginning to have an enormous impact in all areas of society. There were approximately a thousand centenarians in Canada in 2001. By the year 2056, there will be a predicted 63,000 centenarians and, yes, there will be more contenders in the 100+ category for athletic events. In 1993, there were 309,000 people aged 85 and older, and ten years later, in 2013, there were 702,000 people in that group. By the year 2056, there will be almost 2.9 million, which is a 127 percent increase in the over-85 demographic. The UN has estimated that globally, in 2010, there were 765 million people over 60, and by 2050 that number will rise to two billion, with 400 million being over 80 years of age.

The health issues associated with an aging population are not just about the delivery of health services, but the effect they will have on the rest of the community as well. Many family members struggle with raising their own children as well as providing caregiving for elderly parents or relatives, which have many hidden costs. For example, in 2007, employee turnover and missed work due to caregiver obligations cost Canadian employers an estimated $1.28 billion. In that same year, replacing the employees who had to take time off for caregiver obligations cost the economy an estimated $24 billion. An estimated 19 million unpaid hours per week are spent on informal care given to individuals suffering from dementia, and this number will rise to 34 million hours per week over the next 20 years. These costs are both financially and emotionally staggering.

It is essential that caregivers are recognized for the valuable community service they provide when looking after their family members. Also, preventive measures need to be put in place to encourage exercise and socialization outside of caregiving. Each one of us has the ability to look after our own health so we are not an unreasonable burden on our family members. And the number one way to reduce the effects of aging is to get moving. Exercise is key, and secondary to exercise is remaining a part of the community. One of the ways to accomplish being connected to a community is to stay in the workforce. The good news is that with fewer young people available to work, more workers will be needed. Everyone can benefit from a sense of belonging, but unfortunately, the stats are telling a bleak story about social interaction. According to Statistics Canada, 24 percent of the population retires early because they suffer from three or more chronic health conditions. I think the picture is pretty clear and tells us that we all need to take more responsibility to look after our health. This needs to happen right away.

Numbers and statistics tell a story of the past, but at this moment, we can start imagining a different story with a happy outcome. This idea of an age-friendly community has always been near and dear to my heart and is one area of focus during my public presentations on the importance of a healthy community. The best part of making small town or large urban centers senior friendly is that the benefits extend to younger families. For example, walkways and public washrooms designed for accessibility not only benefit the elderly but are essential components for a child-friendly community as well.

My community of Salt Spring Island has many examples of poor planning, including a lack of suitable infrastructure and facilities for young families and seniors. There are no paved walkways around the community of Ganges for those who need a walker or stroller. Many of the parking spots are on an incline without a step up to a sidewalk for easy access. The public bathrooms are not wheelchair friendly, nor do they include a change station for babies.

There is a decided lack of benches around Ganges for those who need to have a rest. Many stores are inaccessible for walkers and strollers. A nice flat paved walkway is nonexistent for those who wish to have a stroll, but don't want to have to be confined to a parking lot.

The mean population here on our island is closer to 55 years while the Canadian average is 40. After taking the time to research our local government (the Islands Trust), our provincial representative (MLA), and our federal representative (MP), a clear vision for Salt Spring and the creation of age-friendly physical and social environments is not apparent to me. The areas that need focus in order to support our seniors are outdoor spaces and buildings, transportation and housing, ongoing respect and social inclusion for all ages, not only seniors, and opportunities for employment. Many seniors would stay in the workforce if they had more flexibility with their work schedule, and if they lived in an age-friendly environment.

Communication and information need to be adjusted as many older people become disconnected from society as technology evolves. Many seniors have never used the Internet, still use land lines, and don't understand why their younger relatives never call. Even our local hospital does not have Wifi access, making it extremely difficult for recovering patients to keep up with the outside world. In addition, there is a strong need for community support services and health services to assist with seniors, particularly those who want to remain at home. If our local politicians, MLA or MP, do not address these issues, then it's time to apply some pressure in order to have these needs recognized. This is particularly relevant at a time when over half of all government spending will be on healthcare.; Costs are spiraling upward, but the quality of life certainly is not.

The Gym Is the New Health Care Center

In the introduction to this book, I mentioned that a gym is a social club as well as a fitness club. My hope is that, in the future, there will be a continued emphasis on exercise as the best way to slow down the effects of aging, increase enjoyment of life, and provide a sense of social inclusion and activity for all ages. Fitness or recreation centers will certainly play a strong role in creating a healthier community, including a healthier group of seniors. If a person is severely deconditioned, of course, special care is required with exercise selection and equipment choice. A good example of creating a healthy community is in injury prevention, namely preventing falls. One of the biggest costs in healthcare is incurred when a senior citizen falls, suffers a fracture, and must spend an extended period in a hospital bed. A hip fracture can take up to ten weeks to repair with the patient spending a large chunk of that time in acute care.

Preventing falls involve reducing drug interactions as well as individuals working on maintaining their balance. At my gym, I stressed to my clients that balance is lost as we get older if we stop challenging ourselves because of fear and inactivity. Balance practice is best carried out in a safe environment like a fitness center with equipment that allows for progressive exercises. We must also adopt the understanding that we have to use balance skills or we will lose balance skills.

Currently, Health Canada predicts that Canadians will sustain somewhere between 2.1 to 3.1 million falls in the year 2036. Proper exercise selection and physical environments designed to reduce the likelihood of falling could reduce the number of predicted falls by as much as 50 percent according to the Ministry of Health. If the total cost of fractures were reduced, there would be more funding available for education, better community recreation facilities, and programs to reduce poverty.

The takeaway message is that everyone's health matters in a community. Older, healthier citizens do not necessarily cost the healthcare system. Unhealthy people at any age are a burden that cannot be sustained by the taxpayer indefinitely. It is said that it takes a whole community to raise a child, but it takes a whole – and holistic – community to look after all its members. One of the reasons that Salt Spring Island has an active, thriving population is the attention people pay to their health and the health of the planet. Finding community at the gym means physical, emotional, and spiritual health.

Be a part of creating the community you wish to live in, one exercise at a time.

11:

Exercise Your Brain. Family and Friends Will Miss You When It's Gone

The most important organ we have is our brain, an organ that has been largely ignored in scientific research over the last hundred years, thanks to the conclusions drawn by Nobel Prize winner Santiago Ramón y Cajal who wrote in 1913 that "adult brain pathways are fixed and immutable." He suggested that "the cells of the brain die as we age and nothing may be done to regenerate the brain."

Then, in 1998, a researcher named Fred Gage teamed up with Swedish neuroscientist Peter Eriksson and completed a study that was published that same year in *Nature Medicine*. The research project, carried out on older Swedish cancer patients, demonstrated that even adult human brains could produce new neurons. These newly formed neurons were located in the hippocampus (a part of the brain associated with memory), proving that it retains its ability to generate new neurons throughout life.

WHY IS THE RESEARCH IMPORTANT?

At one time, scientists and medical doctors believed that a brain would wither up and stop working over time. For most of human history, people have held this belief, and considering the inevitability of our brains shrinking and bodies falling apart, giving up and hitting the rocking chair on the front porch just seemed appropriate. But then something happened! In addition to Gage and Eriksson's revolutionary research, dramatic increases in technology, access to nutritional food, improved sanitation, immunizations, and improved pre-natal care meant that people started to live longer. Longevity is a fact. It's no longer *what if I live a long life*, but *what will I do with the extra 20 to 30 years?*

After the 1998 research on older Swedish cancer patients, research on the brain has started to reveal many interesting facts about the plasticity and cognitive abilities well into old age. In addition, people have become more concerned with brain health as they realize that they are living longer and that the health of their brain is no longer only about age. As the population grows older, people are starting to pay more attention to the increase in diseases like dementia and Alzheimer's disease. Watching relatives and older friends suffer the effects of dementia is enough to set off alarm bells.

Many of us assume, as I used to, that dementia was just a normal part of aging, but that is not true. Research has proven that age may be a risk factor for dementia, but there are many other factors involved with this condition, the biggest of which is a lack of exercise. There are measures we can take to protect the brain, such as maintaining a healthy diet, doing puzzles and brain teasers such as crosswords and Sudoku, reading regularly, keeping up with a stimulating social environment, moderating alcohol and drug consumption, and sustaining a loving long-term partnership. None of these activities, however, protect the brain as much as exercise.

In my opinion, one of the best books about aging gracefully is *What Makes Olga Run: The Mystery of the 90-Something Track Star and What She Can Teach Us About Living Longer, Happier Lives* (2014) by Bruce Grierson. In the book, Grierson writes, "If Sudoku puzzles are a snow shovel, then exercise is a bulldozer." The good news is that if you combine all factors to protect your brain with exercise you get more than $1+1=2$. You get $1+1=5$. Olga, the subject of Grierson's book, is quoted as saying, "Exercise does not add years to your life, but adds life to your years."

BRAIN 101

The average brain weighs about three pounds and is home to approximately 100 billion neurons and 100,000 miles of blood vessels. Our brain uses 20 percent of our oxygen at rest and is composed of 75 percent water. While we are awake, our brains generate 10 to 23 watts of power, which is enough energy to power a light bulb.

Excessive stress can alter brain cells and their functions. The brain is also the host of our mind, which, when active, sends signals through the central nervous system that create movement in our bodies. About 90 percent of what we do happens unconsciously. The rest of the time we have to reason, plan, assess, analyze, and pay attention to our emotions and behaviors. This type of thinking, remembering, learning, and engaging is called cognition or cognitive function, and research on the effects of exercise on the brain can be measured by changes in cognition. A good example is a paper published in 2006 by researchers Kramer, Erickson, and Colcombe entitled, "Exercise, Cognition, and the Aging Brain." They examined the effects of various physical activities on the brain to measure positive effects on cognition. They basically found out that our brains respond to exercise in a very positive way.

Apparently, we have an area in our brain called the executive central command. This area seems to be most affected by exercise, and additionally, is protected by exercise. This central command area is responsible for working memory, planning, scheduling, multitasking, and dealing with doubt and uncertainty. Many may recognize this as an area that slows down as we age or when we are under increased stress such as when we remember that a coffee cup is on the roof of the car as we drive away or we lose our keys or forget appointments and names. This is a gradual slowing down, but as it −turns out, if we exercise regularly, we improve our central command unit. The trick is to ramp up our motivation and adhere to a regular exercise routine.

EXERCISE ADHERENCE, MOTIVATION, SELF-EFFICACY AND THE BRAIN

Researchers who study human behavior know that self-efficacy ("I have confidence in my ability to exercise and stick to it"), feelings of self-worth ("I am worthy"), and eating a healthy diet are directly related to adhering to a program. When you tell yourself that you are going to our personal training session because "I want to, it makes me feel good, and I am worth the time," your chance of success in maintaining a lifestyle change is good.

The other conditions for exercise compliance include a supportive environment, guidance from a knowledgeable fitness professional, support from a significant other or close friend, and access to a safe and user-friendly facility. Watching others exercise while working out proves to be very motivating as well. When you stick to an exercise routine, all the positive changes to your brain are realized, reinforcing your desire to carry on with your fitness-oriented lifestyle. Not only will that command center be better at planning and reasoning, there will also be new connections growing in the dentate gyrus (a small section of the hippocampus that is crucial for memory). New blood vessels will form in the brain for more efficient oxygen transport and waste removal so there will be less garbage to slow down your thinking.

There is also evidence that exercise leads to an increase in the type and quantity of neurotransmitters, chemicals that allow a flow of electric impulses from nerve to nerve. Missing neurotransmitters are like missing the metal prongs at the end of a plug – no electrical conduction will occur. The well reported "runners high" happens as a result of an increase in certain neurotransmitters, and that "high" keeps millions of people running for miles every week. These positive changes to the brain make you feel better and increase your motivation to keep heading back to the gym to maintain these effects.

THERE IS EVEN MORE GOOD NEWS!

Most of the research about the brain and exercise has involved cardiovascular training or aerobics. In 2010, scientists O'Connor, Herring, and Caravalho wrote a paper about the effects of weight resistant training on mental health. They reviewed seven papers that found a reduction of anxiety and an increase in cognition in adults engaged in a weight-training program.

In 2000, a Duke University Study found that weight resistant exercise was better at treating depression than the medication Zoloft. O'Conner et al reviewed eighteen different studies on depression and found that resistance training reduced depression significantly.

Apparently, 25 percent of the US population experiences chronic fatigue. In 94 percent of 70 studies reviewed by O'Conner's team regarding chronic fatigue, the exercise proved to work better than drugs or seeing a psychologist, and strength training, in particular, seems to give the biggest improvement.

When it comes to self-esteem, the paper suggests that strength training will improve the self-worth of younger and older folks and those with cancer and depression.

Even sleep is improved with weight lifting. Lack of sleep can lead to all types of health issues and a generally decreased quality of life. Lifting weight can also lower the risk of sleep apnea. Be patient, though, as it can take eight to ten weeks of consistent weight training to see a difference.

Even people with Parkinson's disease responded to weight training. In a small study published in the *Journal of Applied Physiology*, authors found that after sixteen weeks of three-times-a-week weight training, subjects diagnosed with Parkinson's showed an increase in strength, muscle size and power, and more importantly, an increase in balance, muscle control, cognition, mood, and sense of wellbeing.

Arthur F. Kramer, who was mentioned earlier, is a prominent researcher and expert in the relationship between body fitness and mind fitness. In order to study the effects of moderate activity on the brain, Kramer had a group of sedentary folk (and I mean couch potatoes) between the ages of 60 and 80 start a walking program. They began with fifteen minutes a day and worked up to 45 minutes a day for a six-month period. The results were astounding. The brains of these couch potatoes grew! The hippocampus, frontal, and temporal lobes grew. Not only did the brain show growth, the gray matter (neurons) and white matter (connecting pathways) also increased.

Researchers at Princeton recently found that new neurons built by exercise, in adults, have a dampened response to stressful situations. In other words, neurons built from exercise and sweat are resistant to the stresses and fears that many people begin to experience as they age. Remember the movie *Grumpy Old Men*? They wouldn't have been grumpy old men if they had gotten off the couch and started walking, especially if they had walked fast enough to break a sweat, as it turns out that intensity does matter. Older women seem to respond the most to intense exercise, so as a woman reading this, don't be afraid to sweat and breathe hard. You don't have to go hard every time you exercise. Light activity is better than no activity, but if getting out of a chair is a nine out of ten on your perceived exertion scale, it is time to bump up that effort when exercising.

How Exercise Challenges Can Create Big Changes

Recently, my friend and I started a 30-day squat challenge, thanks to a challenge shared on Facebook. We started with 50 in a row and kept adding squats (with rest days, of course) until we reached 260 squats in a row by the end of the month. My buddy was completely amazed that she agreed to do the challenge and was able to keep up. Excited about her new adventure, she mentioned it at her place of work, and one of her colleagues decided that she and her husband needed to start the challenge. There was a problem. Her husband, a man in his forties with a manual job, could only do 30 squats in a row. It was a typical situation in which a person discovers his poor fitness level. It is usually not until poor health strikes that one realizes this fact, and by this point, most people lose their motivation to push through an exercise program. It was a gift for this man to get a wake-up call and still be healthy enough to get his fitness back. By the time this couple gets to 260 squats in a row, they will both notice many positive changes and hopefully continue on the road of exercise and fitness. The best part is that it is a couple working out together, because as we now know, support of a significant other is very important to exercise adherence.

This chapter has pointed out that increased aerobic fitness and weight resistant training improves memory and cognitive function of the brain. When tests on mice demonstrated that aerobic exercise builds new neurons in the brain, particularly in the dentate gyrus (that small section of the hippocampus responsible for memory) entire science faculties rushed out to buy running shoes. In his book *Buddha's Brain* (2009), Dr. Rick Hanson reveals new scientific research around how our brains and minds work, pointing out how exercise combined with meditation can increase the number of neurons in our brain and create new pathways that reduce stress and increase memory and cognitive function. We have more control over our minds than was previously understood, and when we engage in intense and moderate exercise, we think more clearly, remember more easily, and have an easier time controlling those negative thoughts and angry outbursts.

Just this year, scientists discovered the place in our brains that motivates us to exercise, called the dorsal medial habenula. Scientists went on to knock out the motivation center for exercise in the brains of mice, making sure this center could be reactivated if the mice hit a certain button in their cage. The results of the study revealed that mice chose to activate their motivation center and then run on their exercise wheel. What does this mean? It may be too soon to tell, but I think that we all have a built-in desire to be well and healthy.

Maybe one day there will be a way to activate that motivation center in humans, perhaps by a cell phone Ap. Until then, keep in mind all the great things you are doing for your body and brain every time you pick up that gym bag and hit the cardio equipment, aerobics classes, and weights.

12:

Dieting and Weight Loss–You Can Escape the Quick Sand

This chapter was the most challenging to write. As a professional in the fitness industry, I understand that the subject of weight loss represents many issues for many people. The subject of obesity is primarily about unresolved emotions, but it is also about money, power, and greed. To have a balanced discussion about obesity, there has to be a conversation about agriculture and the food industry. The medical system and government policies need to be included for their contribution to and their vision of overcoming this issue.

There is, of course, a certain genetic component to obesity, but at the end of the day recognizing and managing all contributing factors is the best solution.

What Has Happened to Us Over the Past 50 Years?

I was recently informed that 50 years ago one person out of four would be overweight at a dinner party, but now it is often the opposite with one out of four *not* being obese. There are many contributing factors involved in someone eventually becoming overweight and/or obese. Adults who have a BMI (body mass index) of 25 to 29 are considered overweight while those with a BMI of more than 30 are considered obese. BMI is a measurement of a person's weight compared to their height and should be measured by a physician for the most accurate number.

In terms of the scale of complexity, in which one is the least complex to resolve and a hundred is the most complex, a patient going to see a doctor with a sore throat would be a one and a cancer diagnosis about a 25. A patient presenting with obesity and looking for a solution would be a 99. Dealing with the complex causes, effects, and treatments of obesity is difficult and no easy solution exists. Helping individuals overcome an eating disorder is like pulling them out of quicksand.

There is a huge industry that sells diet pills, books, commercial weight-loss programs, etc., that is aimed at providing a solution. It is a multi-billion-dollar industry that continues to grow daily. Amazon alone has over 33,000 books available to purchase on diet and weight loss. In 2008, in the US, between $33 and $55 billion was spent on weight loss products and services, including medical procedures and pharmaceuticals, with weight loss centers making up about 10 percent of that expenditure.

Canadians have always considered obesity to be an American issue, but the obesity rates in Canada are similar. As mentioned in a previous chapter, there are currently as many morbidly obese people living in Canada as the entire population of Saskatchewan. During the six years that I ran a membership gym, I personally knew three of our members before, during, and after they went into the hospital to have gastric bypass surgery. Even gastric bypass offers no guarantee of success. One of my clients had the surgery and then lost almost 100 pounds, but following the operation, she traveled back east to visit her family where she promptly regained over 20 pounds during the two-week visit, no doubt as a result of emotional triggers.

The quick and easy diets almost always fail, but the drastic surgical interventions don't have a high success rate either. Surgery is a drastic measure and often yields potentially dangerous outcomes. The reality is that even the threat of premature death, discomfort, shame, joint pain, and general loss of enjoyment of life due to obesity is not enough to curb the appetite of 75 percent of the adult North American population.

I first recognized the extent of this problem about ten years ago when I took my two oldest daughters with me on a business trip to an IDEA fit conference in Manhattan. We left from the Seattle Airport. My middle daughter, Monique, who was 13 at the time, had a quiet manner that belied her quick, resourceful mind. The three of us were among the first to board the airplane and find our seats. As Monique sat down to take the middle seat she paused and looked at the passengers wandering into the cabin of the airplane. She turned to me, and in a rather loud voice said, "Mom, what do you think the weight limit is for each seat on this airplane?" Immediately following that comment, the woman in front of us made a request for a seat belt extender from the flight attendant.

None of us really want to engage in this conversation, no matter what our individual size or health status. It is an awkward and sensitive subject that all of us, in some way, can relate to. However, as a former gym owner and a trainer in the trenches trying to keep my clients out of the fat war, I feel that it is important to give my perspective and help to offer some solutions to this ubiquitous problem. There are so many emotional issues around food and body image, and just asking people to follow a textbook formula never felt right to me. Once again, there needs to be a holistic approach to health and fitness. There needs to be an approach inclusive of mind/body and spirit.

UNDERSTANDING WEIGHT LOSS IS BEGINNING TO CHANGE WITHIN THE PERSONAL TRAINING COMMUNITY

Fulfilling my vision to become a more knowledgeable personal trainer involved taking a course on something called muscle activation technique (MAT). It is a massage technique that involves testing for muscle weakness and then pressing on the muscle where it attaches to the bone. It sounds simple, but as there are over 200 muscles in the body, it is anything but simple. Remembering the muscles' names, locations, and what they do anatomically requires involved study and practice. It also means touching people's bodies and sometimes causing them discomfort, even if it is just for a few moments.

Part of the process of this technique was for me to learn a whole new love of the human body. *Every Body is Beautiful* has become one of my mantras. Spending time working with people who were in pain due to the muscular imbalance caused me to rediscover a new respect for the body. We are ultimately energy bodies whose manifestation in concrete form is a way of moving energy around within a physical world. Our bodies get out of sorts because we either trap or scatter energy through overuse, stress, and injury, and then a pain syndrome develops and further complicates the free flow of energy and creates a whole other set of problems.

When we restrict movement to avoid pain, it causes other muscles and joints to become imbalanced and further pain syndromes can manifest. The brain's natural reaction is to stop the painful joints from moving, which can reduce fitness and lead to weight gain. The cause and effect get mixed up and a person can feel like a dog chasing its tail. It was not unusual to meet a client who had been through months, if not years, of different treatments, trying to get relief from physical pain and discomfort.

This same vicious cycle occurs, not just when facing pain and reduced fitness levels, but also when dealing with weight gain and obesity. The more money and time we spend trying to deal with the obesity epidemic, the more money and time we spend dealing with the obesity epidemic. Then, there is the entire diet and dieting quagmire. When I think of dieting to lose weight, I immediately have an image of quicksand. I visualize a slightly overweight individual choosing to go on a diet as if they are choosing to step into the quicksand that lies in their path, rather than going around it. They lose some weight and can move a little easier to nearly climb out of the quicksand, but when they return to their usual diet, they quickly gain back all the weight, and often a little extra. Now they sink a little deeper into the quicksand and it becomes urgent to find a quicker, more drastic way to lose weight, such as restricting caloric intake to less than 1000 calories a day.

They become light enough to move through the quicksand, searching carefully for solid ground. Just before they regain their footing, all the effort of simply climbing out has them exhausted and they pause in their journey. They end up binge eating and drinking, gaining all the weight back, plus another 30 pounds this time.

Now they sink right up to their necks and complete desperation sets in. Desperate people will do desperate things. Maybe they will consider a vacation to a supervised spa where they will eat carrot sticks and celery for a month. Maybe they will choose to get vitamin B shots in their bottom every day and eat prepackaged food endlessly until the weight shifts. There is always a chance to audition to get a spot on reality TV's *The Biggest Loser*, sweating for eight hours a day while a trainer screams at contestants until the weight is gone. At the end of it all, when a person stops being hyper-vigilant even for a moment, the weight comes back like an avalanche, crushing the body and spirit. Finally, the quicksand takes over the whole body and the struggle ends. The body is another statistic, another failure.

Unfortunately, with the evidence removed from the public eye, the dieting drama can continue, unchecked by rational thought or common sense. Privacy and taboo issues that often accompany obesity need to be discussed openly without shame or blame. If a person fails to lose weight, they should not be disregarded or considered a failure. Rather, different approaches need to be considered. There needs to be a solid path built through the quicksand.

A QUIET REVOLUTION

As the weight loss industry booms and the creation of elaborate weight loss schemes becomes a fixation of both experts and consumers, a quiet revolution is happening. It is a whisper that is becoming louder as it gathers more energy and speed. The new path to health is about changing the way we think about weight, food, and health. It is a holistic approach that is both humane and compassionate.

The first whisper of this new sanity was in a book lent to me by my good friend Wendy Giffen, called *The Gabriel Method* (2008) by Jon Gabriel. The book is a must-read for everyone, whether you are at your ideal weight or not. I recommend this book because Gabriel describes the emotional and psychological causes of obesity, creating a universal empathy for the everyday struggle of those who need to deal with their weight. I am not overweight, and except for a few brief occasions in my life when I put on an extra five to ten pounds, I have never been overweight. Even through my four pregnancies, I gained only 25 pounds during each and lost the weight within a month of each birth. However, I come from a family of overweight and obese individuals. My mom, when she was at her heaviest, at five-foot-four, ended up tipping the scales at almost 200 pounds in her mid-fifties. Her mother, my grandmother, was always about 100 to 150 pounds over her ideal weight, and my father and his siblings have struggled with their weight for as long as I can remember. At one point, my Dad was about 70 pounds heavier than he should be for his height and bone structure. To this day, he still talks about needing to lose weight.

When people meet me, they assume that I have good genetics, but that is not at all the case. What I do have, according to Jon Gabriel, is a mental and emotional life that creates an environment for maintaining a healthy weight. After reading *The Gabriel Method*, I developed an even deeper compassion for those who struggle with their weight. I believe everyone needs to be compassionate and loving towards themselves and others in this struggle.

It is important to keep in mind that the struggle is emotional and mental. It is not just about food. Poor quality food in abundance at low prices has just made the emotional and mental struggle more obvious. When I was a small child, I observed with fascination the relationship my adult relatives had with food. Even as a youngster I knew that there was something wrong and deeply emotional about their excessive consumption of calories. When I was full I left the table, but I watched the adults continue to indulge. Even though I was young and could not fully interpret the situation, something did not seem right.

As a personal trainer, I have observed this same food addiction in some of my clients. No matter what I said or preached to my clients, nothing changed. This continually perplexed me until I came to understand the emotional aspects of their condition. With every hurt feeling, anxious feeling, and feeling of unworthiness comes the urge to protect oneself. Food is then consumed and metabolized into fat storage. Every overweight client had the same story.

Not having the right language to speak to this realization, I decided to help them at least focus on the positive effects of exercise, even if weight loss did not occur immediately.

Some clients had success just being in a supportive, non-judgmental environment, and for others, just being able to exercise without joint or muscular pain was enough to get them back on track to lose those extra pounds.

My staff and I made a decision very early on that we were not a weight loss clinic, but exclusively a health and fitness center. We made it clear to our clients that weight was not the measurement that mattered at the outset, but that what mattered was deciding to get healthy and to start a life-long journey of health and fitness. When clients wanted to focus on weight loss and were open to options other than dieting, I recommended both emotional and nutritional counseling.

BOOKS AND ADVICE ARE CHANGING PEOPLE'S BELIEFS

Another book that joins the quiet revolution against the insanity of dieting is Marianne Williamson's *A Course in Weight Loss (2010)*. Like Gabriel, Williamson looks at the emotional basis of weight gain. Both books offer diet-free methods of transformation. This approach will slowly take hold and, within a few decades, this era of obesity will be looked on as a time in history where humans began to transform their minds and their bodies.

Along this line of thinking, diets need to become a thing of the past and the growing and delivery of food need to change to a system of sustainability and sustenance. The film *Just Eat It*, produced by a young couple named Jen and Grant, in Vancouver, BC, is gathering a large following as people become interested in revolutionizing our food industry. This film is a must-see, as it is one of the most informative and thought-provoking films about our food industry that I have ever watched. The film is a reminder of how much we all over-consume with disregard to the effects on our beautiful planet.

As a result of an increasing public awareness, restaurants will prepare food differently and the selection of food on the menu will change. The entire dieting industry will slowly dwindle down to a very small niche as children are educated on the necessity of consuming healthy foods and the benefits of exercise.

I remember being at a restaurant about ten years ago on Salt Spring Island, where two women at the next table were discussing the Zone Diet versus the Atkins Diet. I could not help but overhear their conversation and think to myself about all the hype around diets and how distracting it is, as the real issues get buried and stored away. I remember thinking that such discussions need to change to a conversation of health and fitness pursuits. I was disappointed by the comments on the perceived value of dieting and wanted to reach out and discuss the need to focus on how we are living a life of health and the best ways to look after our planet and its population.

There are a few dedicated individuals who have lost weight and kept it off. The website for the National Weight Control Registry (NWCR) keeps track of more than 10,000 people who have lost weight and successfully kept the weight off for five or more years. The NWCR was developed in 1994 to identify and investigate the characteristics of individuals who successfully maintain weight loss. The registry consists of 80 percent women and 20 percent men. The average age of the women is 45 with an average weight of 145 pounds. The averages for men are 49 years and 190 pounds. Registrants report an increase in energy and physical mobility, better mood, increased self-confidence, and overall improved physical health after the weight loss.

Participants are required to fill out surveys and their condition is tracked on a regular basis. The individuals who have had success have the following behaviors:

- 98% modified their food intake
- 94% increased their physical activity
- 78% eat breakfast
- 75% weigh themselves once a week
- 62% watch less than ten hours of TV per week
- 90% exercise for an average of one hour per day

In every case, there was a turning point at which the person started a journey of achieving and maintaining a healthy weight. The registrants report that losing the weight was more challenging than keeping it off and it seems that some lose the weight quickly, but for others, it is a long process. It is not food intake alone that will create an environment of success. Exercise is essential for weight loss. Every single time an overweight patient or client presents their weight as a concern, they need to be reminded by their healthcare provider that long term successful weight loss is linked to exercise and modified food intake for the remainder of their life.

A NEW APPROACH IS NEEDED

In the first chapter of this book, I mentioned that simply going to the gym does not guarantee weight loss. This is because weight loss requires both an emotional transformation as well as a physical transformation. However, if losing weight is going to be successful, and by success I mean keeping the weight off, daily exercise is going to be essential. Exercise alone can create feelings of wellbeing. Even Jon Gabriel soft sells the idea of exercise in his book because he understands how resistant people are to it. The poor attitude towards exercise will also need to shift in order for people to experience success in maintaining ideal weight and long-term health. It has been my experience that, once a person makes one positive change in their lifestyle such as exercising moderately every day, they will start to look at changes in other areas.

This new paradigm of emotional and physical transformation will need support from elected leaders in all organizations. Once our government policymakers shift to proactive efforts instead of Band-Aid solutions, there will be a monumental shift in our consciousness. Government money saved on fighting the fat war with diets, pills, and surgeries would be better served by funding education, federal income tax credits for fitness memberships, and adequately funded community programs to help those with mental health issues as well as support for those left with emotional difficulties as a result of abuse.

The obesity epidemic is a result of many complex issues and finding the solution does not lie in war. The war on fat is not working because throwing money at Band-Aid solutions is not the answer, and eventually, this struggle will also end as a peaceful solution of compassion as caring and education take over. With this paradigm shift, a change in how we view funding will occur and many individuals can look forward to moving from quicksand to higher, firmer ground.

13:

The Evolution of Energy

"Everyone who is seriously involved in the pursuit of science becomes convinced that a spirit is manifest in the laws of the universe-a spirit vastly superior to that of man." - Albert Einstein, German Theoretical Physicist

Ironically, Bruce Grierson, author of *What Makes Olga Run*, came to Salt Spring Island just as I was beginning to write this chapter. Of course, I was thrilled to attend this presentation knowing that his book is a groundbreaking book about aging and the current scientific understanding of aging. During the question period, a man at the back of the room was commenting in a negative way about the research on exercise and aging and felt that Olga, the subject of Grierson's book, was lucky to have all the stars lined up for her. The man missed the point of the book and Bruce's message in writing the book.

Olga had a deep belief in a power greater than herself and somehow, she understood that her body was simply a vehicle to transport her through her life, but her soul was the fuel to keep the machine moving. Soul, spirit, or energy is the fuel. We can make it a long-lasting resource or let it run out prematurely, but ultimately, we choose. How we get to soul or energy is a personal choice, but is our choice whether we like or not. Even if we keep trying to play the blame game, we still can't escape this universal truth.

Another incredibly positive and empowered woman is entrepreneur Arlene Dickinson, author of *All In (2013)*. Arlene has created an engaging website for entrepreneurs called, https://youinc.com/home where you can find a video posted of an interview with the founder of Goodlife Fitness, David Patchell-Evans. During the four-minute video listed below, David, or Patch, tells us that we need to feel good in our skin, then we need to do things that make us stretch that skin. And above all, we need to stay healthy and fit to be able to do the first two things. https://youinc.com/content/leadership/game-changer-profiles-david-patchell-evans-ceo-founder-goodlife-fitness

The comments from the man at the back of the room during the book discussion would have been entirely different if he knew that he was okay, that his dreams and desires mattered, and he was able to express being inspired by Olga, the 90-year-old track and field star, to stay healthy and fit to accomplish these desires. The conversation would not have focused on his bad knees, aching hips, and other reasons that prevented him from pursuing his dreams.

There is a growing understanding of how exercise and fitness can create the energy to fill that machine to keep it going and purring like a kitten. There is a relevant quote by Neville Goddard, Barbadian author and mystic, which states, "Man's chief delusion is his conviction that there are causes other than his own state of consciousness." Finally, humanity is at the start of removing that delusion.

WHAT IS THIS EVOLUTION OF ENERGY AND WHAT DOES IT HAVE TO DO WITH GYMS AND EXERCISE?

As a personal trainer, I started to see common traits among my successful clients. For those people that came to see me and immediately gave up, nothing in their life changed. If I saw them years later, they would seem heavy and dense, not light and joyful. If they spoke to me, they would be giving the same excuses and the same negative language around their poor health and fitness. As many as 30% of all individuals who walked into the gym to buy a membership or personal training would ask questions and book a session, only to never to be seen again. Those of us in the business were incredulous that exercising could promote so much anxiety and concern. For those of us who treat exercise like brushing our teeth, just a regular thing you do to stay healthy, it seems strange that it is such a major effort to start a regular fitness routine.

In complete contrast, there were the people who would bounce into the gym with the intention of making exercise a part of their life. They just knew that they wanted to get started and were willing to make it a lifelong commitment. Experience is the best teacher, and as I spent more time in my business observing peoples' habits, I was able to better understand what was really happening.

When you are working closely with customers and staff, as I was, in a very personal and intense relationship, awareness begins to increase. This is a wonderful spin-off benefit of being in a people-centered profession. When working with clients, I was privy to their amazing life stories and I also answered questions about my own life and family background. Questions about how and why I became a business owner and/or trainer were frequently fired at me. During these conversations, I would reflect on my own family and I came to realize that no one in my entire family, both immediate and extended, had ever started their own business, or had more than one house at a time, or had been through more than a few long-term relationships.

I think out of all 15 cousins, I was one of four who had ever been divorced. This is a very low percentage considering the average divorce rate is now over 50 percent. I often wonder why I am so different from everyone in my family, standing out like a sore thumb with the acquisition of multiple houses, starting my own business from scratch, and having had many diverse love interests. I am generally excluded from most family gatherings. Perhaps I am considered a danger to the impressionable younger generation?

This theme of being different will be recognizable to the people who choose to make health a priority or have a burning desire to make the world a better place. We individuals stand out and have to clear our own path through the jungle of bad habits and social pressure. The ability to persevere has to do with attitude and a lot to do with an evolving sense of energy and the importance of maintaining positive energy to stay in good health.

HEALTH IS BECOMING THE NEW GREEN

The impact of having access to information, and the realization of potential damage caused by humans to the planet, has started this awareness in choosing how we use our energy and where we direct it. Many people are becoming aware that their choices are having a far-reaching effect on the planet, both positive and negative. There is an old saying that if you are not part of the solution then you are part of the problem. Energy can be directed for the highest good, or not, and evidence of this is painfully obvious if you watch the evening news.

I began my career in the fitness business because I had a vision of health and fitness for my community, my family, and myself. The idea that people lie around in Lazy Boy chairs endlessly watching TV was (and still is) painful to me. I knew the positive energy I would create if I could encourage even a few of my clients to walk in the woods after dinner or ride a bike on the weekends, instead of sitting and engaging in mindless activities. Then I started to read and research extensively on exercise, human behavior, and the physics of energy. As a self-proclaimed research junkie, I left almost no stone unturned in my quest for knowledge. The correlation between people's behavior around their health and the way they view the world became increasingly evident to me as I pursued further understanding.

Scientific research has changed over the last twenty years. We have a whole new concept of the brain and its ability to change, referred to as neuroplasticity. There is an increasing body of evidence about the benefits that gratitude has on our health. Relationships are a huge factor in maintaining health and surviving illnesses like cardiovascular disease and cancer. Volunteering has been shown to improve longevity and boost the immune system. Even meditation is getting more attention and is recognized as a way to improve health and overall enjoyment of life. There are many books being published by scientists and medical doctors like Deepak Chopra, Judith Orloff, Bruce Lipton, Henry S. Lodge, Barbara Brennan, and Rick Hansen to name a few. All of these authors are discussing, in a meaningful way, energy and its effect on the mind and body. Conversations about health and fitness can no longer be separate from conversations about energy and emotions.

WHEN PAIN AND INJURIES ARE YOUR FRIENDS

Those who are successful in living a healthy life find opportunity in illness and injury. Certain injuries that presented at my gym conveyed distinct emotional issues. The shoulders are a target of many pain syndromes and potential injuries. Because the shoulder joint is so flexible in its range of motion, it is particularly vulnerable to overuse and acute injuries, however, there is a certain resistance to joy as evidenced in those who have chronic shoulder pain. The neck is another area affected by stress, especially relationship stress. Many of my clients would arrive at the gym with a very stiff neck and subsequently admit to being in a stressful relationship. The feet and ankles are about the fear of being stable or lack of stability. Over the years, I witnessed many foot issues being resolved when clients practiced balancing and became confident about their ability to stand firm, even in unstable environments. The shooting pain down a leg is usually feeling dead emotionally or having issues around sexuality; the infamous piriformis muscle pain (deep in the buttocks and often referred to as sciatica pain) was a usual complaint when reviewing a member's health history. I have literally witnessed people dragging their leg along behind them in public with visible pain in their face and when asked if they are okay the response would be "Oh I am just getting over this little back thing." Often, I would bite my tongue because I knew how certain exercises along with energy healing could make it so much better for that individual.

Not everyone is ready to make the leap of faith to understand that their body is their friend and wants to be healthy, but often times a little assistance is needed along the way. The greatest part of helping people to overcome their fears and begin exercising as they recovered from an injury or illness was to watch them discover and really feel their bodies for the first time in years or maybe ever.

These individuals would learn correct lifting techniques. They would allow the flow of energy through their bodies and experience the healing that energy would bring. The flow of oxygenated blood to damaged joints creates a healing environment. Muscles that have been neurologically turned off will start to work with correct exercises and a supportive environment. Often, that was enough for pain to disappear quickly without needing drugs. Once a person's fear is gone, and the blood is flowing through their body, they can think more clearly and react in a more logical, rational way. Our thoughts create an impact on our bodies and can create the same suffering as the pain from an acute injury. Every time we act in anger, judge others, seek revenge, or have unkind wishes against others, we experience subtle damage to our bodies that over time can become a full-blown pain syndrome.

There is also such a thing as being a good customer and a good pupil. Those people that came to the gym with a negative attitude and blamed us for failing to achieve their exercise goals did not improve their health and did not enjoy a potentially great experience. For positive energy flow, it is important to be a courteous customer and to have faith and trust in the process of healing and getting healthy. If you don't feel right in a certain place or situation, simply walk away and let it go, but keep looking to find the right space to heal and get physically healthy.

FINDING HEALTH CAN TRANSFORM LIVES

Through the process of living a healthy life, there is an opportunity to discover what you may be missing in your life. Many cancer survivors have left jobs and relationships to pursue their dreams and then gone into remission. If your job is causing you to battle with overuse injuries, it may be time to look at other career options. Maybe your body is telling you to grab that camera and take those photos you have been dreaming about. Many people who have jobs where they sit all day decide to quit that job and take up occupations where they can move around more and do what they love to do. Some people have left the cubicle to start a career where they work hands-on with others and are not tethered to a computer day in and day out. I knew a woman in her 50s that went back to school to become a nurse after her children left home. She fulfilled her dream of helping others.

There are those who give up secure jobs to take up organic farming because they know the stress of their career is killing them. Working with soil and being connected to the earth is healthy energetically and satisfying. Knowing that you are growing wholesome organic food that will contribute to the health and wellbeing of others is deeply satisfying for some.

EXPERIMENT WITH YOUR ENERGY FLOW

The flow of energy that goes into the world from healthy, happy bodies has a multiplying effect. Try this small experiment to witness this effect: for six months, exercise regularly; appreciate everyone who is exercising with you or around you; post positive comments on your Facebook page about exercise and your exercise buddies; tell everyone that they are worth the benefits of becoming fit; thank the instructors, personal trainers, and employees at your fitness facility, and tell your family that you know they are worth it every single time they do something healthy.

Let the people you work with know that you are manifesting a healthy life and that they are also worthy of a healthy, engaged life. Ask those around you if you can help them to begin an exercise program or motivate them to adhere to a program. Every day when you wake up, express gratitude to be alive; for the opportunity each day to take care of your body in order to enjoy life to its fullest. After six months of doing these things, you will notice a change in yourself and those around you. You will make new friends and feel happier and more connected to yourself and others.

We have evolved from single-celled organisms to multi-celled organisms in a relatively short space of time. At one time, not so long ago, we lived in caves and every day was a struggle for survival. Now, there are 7 billion people on the planet, when 40 years ago scientists swore up and down that earth could not support more than a few billion.

Our ability to communicate has exploded with the invention of computers, the Internet, and social media. Technology has given us a longevity bonus of an extra 20 to 30 years of life. There is an increasing awareness of how we use our energy and how our actions affect everyone. Our survival and evolution will depend on how we look after our bodies, minds, and soul. I am hopeful and excited about the endless possibilities ahead for human beings and hope that my message inspires you to join in with this evolution towards positive, healing energy.

14:
Final Thoughts

As I begin to write this final chapter, my heart is whispering gratitude to me. There are many things to be grateful for, but in this moment, I feel enormously grateful that the events of my life have lined up to allow me an opportunity to put pen to paper. As many of you will relate, life is never totally easy or smooth sailing. The winds come up, sometimes unannounced in the middle of the night, waking us from a peaceful sleep. At other times, the doldrums strike and we go nearly mad with impatience, deeply desiring some kind of movement. The one constant thread throughout my life has been a joy and love of physical movement. Watching others find and embrace that joy has filled my soul with boundless energy year in and year out. Most of us have moments in our life that are true game changers. I recently had my game changer, my scare, my health challenge, and it provided me with that rare opportunity to really deeply contemplate my life's true purpose.

In the fall of 2014, I decided to drive to Calgary for a job interview and to visit my son Luc at the same time. Before I left, I announced to my friends that I was seriously considering a move, not only for financial reasons and career opportunities but maybe for an adventure as well.

My business had sold and I was feeling directionless so off I went to see the mountains on my way to Cow Town. It was October 1st, the day before my birthday, and it turned out to be a day I will never forget. While I was driving, a message came through on my cell phone from my family doctor. I pulled over to listen to the message, which was to inform me that results had come back from an analysis of a mole I'd had removed from the back of my leg and that I needed to call the doctor immediately. It was the end of the day and I knew I would not be able to contact the doctor's office until the next morning. I took a deep breath and continued driving through the night along winding mountain roads, negotiating a blizzard that seemed to come from nowhere, and mentally writing my eulogy.

After what seemed like hours, I reached my destination and settled in for the night. As I lay in bed staring up at the hotel ceiling, my heart was pounding in my chest, and for the next eight or so hours, I went deep into my heart and looked honestly at my life. The very first realization I had was that I had no regrets. Even though I'd experienced difficult challenges and moments of despair in my life, I knew in that moment I would not change a thing. The other realization that came to me was my desire to be near friends and loved ones for the rest of my life. Moving to a new place was not what I really wanted. I would have loved to embark on such an adventure, but not at the expense of solid relationships.

While I was in Calgary, I had a wonderful time and I even made some new friends when I went to view an apartment. I made arrangements to meet up with a lovely man that I had met on Salt Spring in the summer, and we caught up over a delicious steak dinner, talking for hours about everything that really matters. My son and his friends took me out for my birthday and I danced all night, feeling twenty again. I did go to the job interview and met a dynamic group of people who spent each day in the trenches, giving their members and clients great service and the benefits of a healthy lifestyle. Just this morning I had an email from the owner of that gym, keeping me updated on the club happenings.

Once I finally reached my doctor by phone, she let me know that the mole was a stage zero melanoma, but I had to be back in BC in a few days' time to see a plastic surgeon. I said my goodbyes and headed back to Salt Spring Island.

During the twelve-hour drive home, I realized that I wanted to pursue my dream of writing a book and becoming a motivational speaker. It also became clear to me that I wanted to remain on Salt Spring and stay connected to my friends and the community that I had called home for seventeen years. A year and a half earlier, I had started to write a book about joining a gym, and now I found myself with the time and motivation to finish that book. Because I was working long hours in my business, I had neglected my health by not finding a new family doctor after my doctor left Salt Spring, and had not been for a checkup in three years. It was only when my business sold that I started to take care of myself, which led me to a wonderful and caring physician who I credit with saving my life. It was a get out of jail free card. I not only met a new doctor who made a connection to me and gave me her unconditional support, but it presented me with the opportunity to reach out to a wider community with the message of fitness and connection to individual purpose.

The plastic surgeon was a vibrant young man named Alex Anzarut. We met on Monday, October 6th, 2014 and established an instant rapport as we chatted about life, wellbeing, and how relationships have a profound effect on health and happiness. Alex showed me his favorite book covers as we discussed my book and what topics it would cover. Instead of a lengthy discussion of moles, cancer, and other medical issues, the majority of our time together was focused on the importance of creating a meaningful life. I promised Alex that I would acknowledge him in my book as he came into my life at a turning point – a place where each of us will eventually arrive, faced with decisions that will alter the course of our future. We will meet people on our journeys who make these choices easier by gently steering us in the direction our hearts have been waiting for. It was not a coincidence that I met two forward-thinking, engaged medical professionals who both desire a rich and meaningful life for their patients. It is with tremendous joy and gratitude that I give my deepest thanks to both Gisella and Alex.

Then, suddenly, the book was written. It is an expression of years of dedicated work in the fitness profession and a result of over fifteen years of connection to clients, members, community, and many dear friends. For years, I wore three hats: the mom hat, the business owner hat, and the landlady hat. Working closely with people has had the most profound effect on my character development, helping me to learn more about compassion, love, and the strength of the human spirit as I became aware of the struggles many people live with on a daily basis. That compassion was essential for me in the gym, reminding me to listen a little closer, and reminding me to care and to connect a little more.

This experience helped me recognize the times when people needed to go, and come back, and when they were ready to embark on a healthy journey. That compassion made me rethink *perfection* and the insanity of chasing an ideal that doesn't exist, except as a method to exploit the vulnerable. At the end of the day, it is the message of compassion, love, and forgiveness that embodies a sense of hope for the future of human beings.

David Patchell-Evans is the founder of the largest chain of gyms in Canada and developed his interest in the fitness business after a nearly fatal motorcycle accident. He states beautifully in a video interview with YouInc, mentioned in a previous chapter, that he wants his legacy to be the knowledge within each individual they are worthy of being healthy, fit, and engaged in life. Those of us fortunate to be a part of the fitness industry hold the same humanitarian philosophy. We know everyone is worthy and deserving of a great life, but it won't happen fully unless we all consider our own personal health, the health of our communities, and the health of the global community. My desire is that somewhere buried in the words of my book is a gentle nudge, a friendly reminder, a whispering resonance that takes you on a healthy, fitness-filled journey towards connecting with your soul's purpose.

May health and happiness follow you to the end of your days.

With all my love,
Sheena

About the Author

Sheena Bull found a passion for exercise when she was fourteen years old and unable to run a mile around the track without stopping during a fitness test. In the month following, she took up a running program and eventually completed the run in 7.5 minutes. She continued to make exercise a part of her life, even during her four pregnancies.

In 1997, Sheena and her family moved to Salt Spring Island, British Columbia, where she created a personal training studio in the back of her home with a treadmill and a few pieces of exercise equipment. Fulfilling a lifelong dream of business ownership, Sheena grew her personal training studio into a full gym with 350 members and a team of four personal trainers.

In 2014, Sheena sold her business and took the opportunity to ride her touring bike from Victoria, British Columbia, to Northern California. During that adventure, she discovered her intuitive side and was inspired to return to Salt Spring Island to write a book about her experiences as a business owner and personal trainer. In her role as an intuitive personal trainer and life coach, Sheena brings her passion for fitness and her love of helping others discover their peak fitness.